# AN INTRODUCTION TO EURYTHMY

# AN INTRODUCTION TO EURYTHMY

*Talks given before sixteen eurythmy performances*

by
Rudolf Steiner

Anthroposophic Press

The sixteen talks presented here were given between 1913 and
1924 in various European cities. The original text of the first talk is
contained in the volume *Die Entstehung und Entwickelung der
Eurythmie* (GA 277a). The fifteen remaining talks constitute a
translation of *Eurythmie als Impuls für künstlerisches Betätigen und
Betrachten*, published by Rudolf Steiner Nachlassverwaltung, Dornach, 1953. All the talks were translated by Gladys Hahn.

**Library of Congress Cataloging in Publication Data**

Steiner, Rudolf, 1861-1925.
An introduction to eurythmy.

Translated from the German.
Talks given between 1913 and 1924 in various
European cities; 15 of the talks constitute a trans-
lation of *Eurythmie als Impuls für künstlerisches
Betätigen und Betrachten.*
 1. Eurythmy—Addresses, essays, lectures.
I. Steiner, Rudolf, 1861-1925. Eurythmie als
Impuls für künstlerisches Betätigen und Betrachten.
English. 1984. II. Title.
BP596.R5S75 1984        793.3'2        84-12263
ISBN 0-88010-042-7

The cover shows the eurythmy figure "Lovable"
by Rudolf Steiner. Lettering by Peter Stebbing.

# Table of Contents

# Introduction

During the years when eurythmy was young and little known, Rudolf Steiner gave nearly three hundred introductory talks about the new art form to a variety of audiences. These talks were full of life and creativity, revealing the richness underlying the spiritual laws of the developing art. Although nearly six decades have gone by since the last of them was delivered, what was spoken at that time can still be as meaningful for readers now as it was for listeners then.

So that we may be stimulated anew by the speaker's words, sixteen of his talks have been carefully selected from the complete collection and are presented here for the first time in English. Since Steiner sought to develop a true feeling for the extraordinary newness of this art, the discussions are more enlightening than explanatory. Directed first only to members of the Anthroposophical Society—later also to the public—he spoke at every opportunity from many different standpoints, often illuminating, with subtle nuance, points previously made.

It was in response to a request for a new impulse in the art of movement, put to Steiner in 1912, that eurythmy took its beginning and the new art was born. Moreover, Marie Steiner was soon drawn into the venture and through her efforts she developed in time the new approach to speech formation and the recitation which is so essential when eurythmy is performed. With this addition performances grew ever more unusual and audiences had to be prepared for their encounters with this wholly new way of presenting drama, poetry and music.

The informality of these little talks should be borne in

mind. They were not meant for publication, but a strong life nevertheless pervades the printed word. Here we find, if we will, the cosmic laws of the new art presented from different aspects. Undoubtedly, what Rudolf Steiner has to say here can be rewarding to those who seek to understand the background of eurythmy.

—Kari van Oordt

January, 1984
Spring Valley, New York

# I

Allow me to make a brief introduction to our eurythmy performance. It seems to be called for because we cannot yet claim any great degree of perfection in our work. So far, it is only an attempt, perhaps only the smallest seed of an attempt. Were I not to say this, one might easily think that we want to compete in our eurythmy with the other arts most nearly related to it, mime and dance, which today are already developed to a high degree of perfection. We are fully conscious of the fact that with this special art form that we are presenting to you, we can offer nothing so finished, so perfected as those neighboring arts. We certainly do not think of ourselves as being in competition with them. Actually, there is no question of our offering anything equal or similar to them. We are involved in something quite different, something new. It rests—as everything does, really, that is cultivated here at the Goetheanum—on Goethe's world conception and on his conception of art. This is not because we want to bring Goethe forward again into our time, but because we feel that his ideas can and must be worked out in relation to the feelings, the artistic and spiritual insights of our modern epoch.

I have no need to speak about our artistic impulse; that you will discover from what you are about to see. It may be important, however, to point out how the particular art form that we call eurythmy actually came into being. I must draw your attention to something that may at first seem theoretical but that is deeply grounded in Goethe's profound view of nature—a view that later developed into his grand conception of art. I am referring to what one calls Goethe's teachings on metamorphosis, which are to be found everywhere in our building transformed into artistic perceptions.

To state it most simply, Goethe saw every leaf, every colored petal as an entire plant. He saw inwardly the process of a single leaf unfolding by metamorphosis into the entire plant; then also by corollary, that the entire plant is only a more complicated leaf.

One can relate Goethe's perception to every living thing, above all to the most complete living thing, man himself. Here in eurythmy it is translated from the world of nature to artistic creation—and not just to the creation of forms but of movements. We are trying to show from intuitive perception the inclinations toward movement, the seeds of movement that are manifest in the human larynx and its neighboring organs when someone speaks—that is, in artistic poetic form —or when he produces musical sounds. At such moments one's attention is directed to what one hears. But if one had some artificial device by which one could see at such a moment how the air mass is stirred to rhythmic vibration by the incipient movements of the larynx and its neighboring organs, he would realize how a whole world arises out of a single human organ complex, how the entire man is revealed through it. Just as a single leaf is metamorphosed into the vastly more complicated form of the whole plant, so in the same way what is perceived intuitively, supersensibly, when someone produces artistic sounds can be transformed into movement and form of the whole man. The whole man can become a larynx. Then what comes to expression in the tiny larynx works in the whole man as significant inner impulses to movement.

Goethe said quite beautifully that art rests on the revelation of nature's secret laws, laws that would never be perceived were it not for art. He said it again from a subjective point of view: "The man to whom Nature begins to unveil her open secret, feels an irresistible longing for her most worthy interpreter, Art." One feels the truth of these words when one transforms what otherwise manifests itself invisibly, supersensibly at the moment of human speech or singing, into movement of the whole human organism.

So what you will see here on the stage is the human larynx made visible in the movements of individuals or groups. Eurythmy is intended to be speech that has become visible. Undoubtedly, art and artistic feeling must provide the entire foundation for the start of eurythmy. What you will see has not arisen from grey theory or science. It is Goethe's conception of nature and art translated directly into feeling. The positions and movements of the individual eurythmists reproduce the inclinations toward movement that are to be seen in the larynx at the moment of artistic speaking or singing. The group movements and the relation of one eurythmist to another reflect the feeling that permeates the speech, the inner attitude of soul, the soul warmth, the attributes one finds in artistic speech such as rhyme, rhythm, assonances, and so on. All that is usually thought of as "style," but thought of only as an audible element, can be expressed visibly by an individual or group in movement. Style, according to Goethe, has to do with the depths of knowledge, with the nature of things, insofar as it is humanly possible to make them comprehensible in visible form. So here we are trying to make the most sublime revelation in the world—man, this microcosm—visible as a great larynx.

I only want to make clear how this art form has arisen. Just as something that nature implants in man can become art—poetry, for instance, or song—so something inherent in the whole being of man can become art. But all I have been saying is only to describe its origin. The artistic element must be left to be experienced through immediate perception, and we are convinced that it can be so experienced.

So we will undertake to bring sound-images to your hearing through the recitation or the music, and at the same time, to your vision through the eurythmy.

Through our recitation also, dear friends, we come into conflict with modern attitudes. Today's young people have not known the old art of recitation, even in its decadence. As late as the seventies or eighties of the past century, its external form was still preserved and cultivated. One needs only to think of Goethe rehearsing his *Iphigenia* in Weimar with a baton. Today there is on the whole no liking for this kind of recitation that is concerned with the form, the truly artistic element. People nowadays value much more the prose content of what is being spoken, and any nuances of meaning that can be emphasized. Here, our recitation must form with the eurythmy a common work of art. We must return —just as the art of the dance needs in many cases to return to the ritual dance of ancient times—so we must return to an earlier style of recitation. Today it is less understood, but it can be understood again even if it comes out of the declining art culture of the nineteenth century, if it will now again contain a fundamental spiritual, supersensible element.

Allow me to close with some words of Goethe from his beautiful essay on Winckelmann. "Since man stands at the summit of Nature, he regards himself also as a complete 'nature' that must produce another summit, this time within himself. To this he climbs by acquiring all perfections and virtues, by decreeing choice, order, harmony, significance and finally by attaining to the creation of works of art that are given a shining place among his other deeds and

4

works.'' One feels the truth of this as one strives here in eurythmy to make the whole man into a work of art.

But for all that, dear friends, I beg you to view what we have undertaken here as no more than the *intention*, as no more than a *beginning*, to reach toward a new art form. We hold a most modest estimate of the level on which our eurythmy still stands. But we believe that from what seems a weak beginning, something really perfect can someday stand forth. Please accept our offering in this sense. We are convinced that the eurythmy we are able to present today will develop—whether it be through us or, if this is denied us, through others—from this small beginning to an independent art that will stand fully recognized beside the other arts.

# II*

We are presenting a new art to you today, but we beg you to realize that this is only its beginning. It will need time to be perfected, but then it will embrace definite and broad purposes. One can already see, even at this elementary stage, what it is intended to achieve for the future of mankind: not to belong to narrow circles of people but to be imbedded in human life, nourishing all of mankind. It is thus intended to fulfill an important task in the future life of humanity.

If I were asked to compare the eurythmy you are going to see here with anything known in the world today, I could not do it. What arts of movement there are, are in each and every case only a part, a piece of what you are about to see. What we are trying to do is to take a few elements essential to a complete human being and pour them together into an activity that will be healthful, invigorating and artistically fulfilling. If I were really put to it to make a comparison, I should have to say that in eurythmy something is striven for in a soul-spiritual way that up to now has been sought for in an *un*soul-spiritual way as, for instance, in gymnastics. There one is brought into bodily movement in accordance with bodily laws. And please to harbor no illusions about it! For gymnastics is an art of movement that contains no soul or spiritual element whatever. By contrast, you will see here an art of movement that lets the soul-spiritual element shine

---

*For the staff and workmen of the Waldorf-Astoria cigarette factory.

7

directly into the movements of the human limbs, letting the eurythmist feel himself as a soul-and-spiritual being.

One could also compare what is offered here with the art of modern dance. That is another one-sided form of artistic movement. Its content is taken from external life; the external world is translated into dance movements.

In eurythmy nothing is taken from external life. What you are going to see are movements of individuals and groups in various relationships of position and movement, all of which you really do yourselves throughout the day! You don't do them with externally visible arms and legs, however, but you *do* do them, nonetheless, whenever you speak. You do them continually with the invisible organs of your larynx and with the air that they set into motion. The fact is simply this, that ordinarily we are not aware of how the larynx and its neighboring organs are vibrating and how the palates and lungs are in movement when we are speaking, how movement is being transformed into sound. If someone were able to see what the larynx, lungs, tongue, palates and lips are really doing, and what the air is really doing during speech, he would say that when we are speaking, beautifully artistic movements are made by all of us, especially during artistic recitation. These artistic movements are similar in their effect to music. Strange as it may seem, this eurythmy that we are presenting has been taken from the secret works of art that every man, even the most ordinary, creates when he speaks.

When an individual eurythmist or a group comes out on the stage, all the individual's movements and the relations of position and movement to one another of a group, everything you see, is transformed movement of the larynx. The entire human being and the entire group you see there are simply a larynx. They have become all speech organ. So we can play music for you and at the same time show you what is in the music, not by movements of the larynx as it would

8

be if we sang, but by eurythmy movements done by groups of eurythmists. So we also can present poetry, artistically formed speech, through the movements of individuals and the movements and positions of groups.

What a single word or sound contains is shown in eurythmy by the movements of an individual, whereas whatever permeates poetic speech with warm human feelings and soul content is expressed by the movements and positions of groups. And all is created in pure rhythm! We can express everything through eurythmy. The part of a man that is most intimately related to his soul, and through which his innermost feelings are made manifest—his organ of speech—is what we carry over in eurythmy to the whole man. We ensoul and inspirit man in eurythmy; we transfer to the spirit what was formed in the body so that he can really experience himself as soul and spirit.

People of our time have forgotten the true art of recitation. No one today recites poetry; they merely read it as prose. Here, we must recognize that poetry is more than just prose. It is structured, molded speech. In our recitation, therefore, we are trying to bring back a truly artistic way of speaking, not the prosaic delivery that is the fashion elsewhere where the artistic element has been lost. Here one recognizes it again when the speakers are also expressing what the eurythmists must express if they are all larynx. You will therefore also be hearing what you are seeing.

So gymnastics, which has no soul, is merged with dance, which has no inner inspiration, and eurythmy is created, something that is not just to be looked at like modern dance and is not just bodily movements like gymnastics, but is both and something new besides. It is an art in which the participant derives health and strength from soul-spiritual sources.

You must realize, however, that this is a large task. Eurythmy is to serve human life in times to come, times of which I spoke to you recently over in the factory from the standpoint of our social problems. It will be able to give new life to liberated human beings if they will take it up with understanding. By that time it will have been perfected, by us or by others. Now it is laying the foundation for the ideal of mankind that must unfold in the future.

# III*

So, dear children! You have come from home to see our beautiful mountains and fields and meadows. And you've found new friends, the kind people who have taken you into their homes. You've been given a warm welcome in this beautiful Switzerland!

Yesterday, we showed you what we are doing up here on the hill. Today, we will show you more of it. There is much for you to see. Perhaps someday you will think back and remember what you saw here; perhaps, also, you will someday understand the word "eurythmy." Then, I hope this present time will be one of your precious memories.

You know that God gave man a most special gift: his speech. Usually people speak with their mouths, don't they? Now, what you have seen here as eurythmy is also speech, but the whole human being is speaking. Someday you will all know what it is that we call the soul of a man. You don't know yet, you can't know, what it is in you that someday you will call "soul."

But what you saw here yesterday, the movements all those people were making with their arms, the movements they were making together in a circle, and everything else they were doing—that was all speech; it was all speaking, though not so that you could hear it. It was speaking so that you could *see* it! And what spoke was not the people's mouths, it was their whole being; it was the soul in them. If

---

*Introducing a program for children on holiday from Munich.

11

someday you wonder, "Does anything live inside me?" the answer will be, "Yes, that's where your soul lives." Remember then that yesterday and today you discovered how a man's soul speaks through him, how it speaks through his arms and legs.

And now I'm going to look right over your heads and say a few words to the grown-ups in back of you, about what you are going to see in a few minutes, which someday you will understand.

I would like to say that our eurythmy—or what we should call our attempt at it—is actually a demonstration of Goethe's world conception, and of his conception of art, not as they were thought of in Goethe's own time, but as we have to think of them in the first third of the twentieth century.

Goethe penetrated more deeply than any of his contemporaries—or any of the generations so far following him—into the living being of nature. The depth of his world conception is even today not yet recognized. This eurythmy of ours, however, should show how his ideas can be applied to a narrow field of work.

Goethe saw a plant, an entire plant, as simply a complicated leaf. For him, every leaf was something in which his supersensible eye saw again the entire plant.

This conception has not even yet been fully worked out. In the realm of art it is capable of much further development. Here, it is being applied to a specific, concrete field.

To one who sees intuitively what takes place in the whole human being when he hears speech, particularly when poetry is recited artistically—to such a person the movements made by the human larynx and its neighboring organs are related to the whole human being in the same way that Goethe saw the leaf to be related to the whole plant; that is, the leaf as a metamorphosis of the whole plant.

To us here, what comes to expression in human speech through the larynx and its neighboring organs is a metamorphosis of what the whole human being is holding back and what he really wants to put into movement when he listens. If one can see supersensibly, one knows that it is more than just a theory when it is suggested that through our speech organs we bring the air into movement. Speech has its own invisible movements, which it carries with it into the air. This is what we are trying to show in eurythmy. We are trying through our movements to make the human being into an enormous larynx, to make perceptible everything that otherwise remains invisible in speech—invisible for the reason that ordinarily a person directs his attention only to what he is hearing with his ears.

To see speech as coming from the whole human being is what we want to achieve by our eurythmy. There is nothing arbitrary about it.

But it has not yet been achieved completely. The art of eurythmy is only at a rudimentary stage. So far, it is only at the beginning of a beginning. All pantomime, anything arbitrary has no place in eurythmy. Just as music has laws, just as one tone follows another from the necessity of a musical law, just as music is structured in major and minor modes from musical laws, so eurythmy is built on inner laws. If two people or two groups of people present the same piece of eurythmy in two different places, there can be no more difference in the separate performances than there can be when two pianists play the same Beethoven sonata with their two personal interpretations. In both instances there is a structure based on laws.

That is what we are striving for, trying thereby first to create something artistic, but also something pedagogical and therapeutic. In our artistic endeavor we must be activated by that broad artistic principle of Goethe's which he expressed in this way: "Since man has been placed at the pinnacle of nature, he sees himself as nature complete, and has again to build up a pinnacle in his own humanity. He rises to this new peak by permeating himself with all perfections and virtues, by calling for choice, order, harmony, meaning, and finally by attaining the creation of works of art, which take a prominent place beside his other deeds and works."

Here, the entire human being becomes a work of art by bringing into play those movements that lie invisible in the whole human being just as they lie invisible in the human larynx. Now they are to become visible.

The glow that illumines someone's speech, coming from the warmth of feeling in his soul, the power that enlivens someone's speech, coming from the enthusiasm of his personality, all that the poet brings to expression through rhyme and rhythm: these things are made manifest by individual movements and group movements in space. This corresponds to inner laws. There is no more subjective element in it than there is in an artistic program when two individuals present one and the same piece of music.

Certainly these introductory words must not encroach upon the artistic program that is coming. After all, true art rests on the fact that it can be enjoyed immediately. Yet, in the sense of Goethe, it should still be pointed out that all artistic creation has a supersensible origin. It is precisely from this source, it seems to me, that we should create a new art form to add to everything else we want to contribute to the Goetheanum.*

The eurythmy will be accompanied by recitation or by music. What we are hearing with our ears will at the same time be presented to our eyes through the eurythmy forms.**

---

*The building in Dornach, Switzerland, designed by Rudolf Steiner and built during World War I and after, as a center for his work. People came from every country to contribute their skills in carving and painting.

**The eurythmy term for choreography.

Here I would like to mention the art of recitation. It must return again to its earlier, good style. People today have really never heard a true art of recitation. That practically ended in the seventies of the last century. Goethe was one person still so permeated by this art of speech that he rehearsed the actors for his play, *Iphigenia*, wielding a baton like a choral conductor. That was quite justified, for in recitation it is not a matter of emphasizing the literal, prose content, as is done today from a certain materialistic tendency, but rather of giving expression to the artistic content, the rhythmic elements, the artistic structure and form. Recitation and eurythmy proceed parallel to each other, and show that it is in the very nature of the human being to move within himself in response to artistic activity.

Remember that Schiller, when he conceived a poem, did not at first hold any literal idea of the poem consciously in his mind, but experienced a vague melody, a musical content in his soul. He created directly out of the musical inspiration in his soul. So at the foundation of his most important poems lies the rhythmic motion, the inner flow, which he then only afterward embodied in a literal content.

We, too, want to leave the prose content of a poem in the background and bring into prominence the truly poetic qualities of the recitations that accompany the eurythmy.

You will realize, of course, that we are only in the very first stage of our eurythmy. Above all, it should be pointed out that pantomime, mime, personal gesture will all have been eliminated when our performance is more perfect. We ourselves are our severest critics. We know that in the art of eurythmy we are still at a level of imperfection. But we believe that in the sense of Goethe's conception, when the whole human being is brought to expression, higher natural laws shine through what is being presented to the external senses. And we believe that on that basis a genuine new art can arise, nobler than any contemporary dance form. Also,

15

in contrast to the current gymnastics, which have only a physiological basis and only build up the external physical body, the movements in eurythmy have a soul origin. There is a soul vibrating, a soul speaking in all eurythmy. Thus, we want to introduce a pedagogical element also into this new art.

I believe we have your understanding for what we will now present to you in such imperfect form. We hope that if our contemporaries respond to these efforts with just the slightest interest, we will be able—perhaps not we ourselves, but those who come after us—to develop this art of eurythmy to such perfection that it will stand beside the other, older arts as a fully recognized new art.

# IV*

One day when Professor Capesius was visiting Felicia Balde, he said that he always felt so refreshed by the stories and fairy tales she told.** Now, Dame Balde is a straightforward person who says exactly what she thinks, so she gave Capesius this answer: "Yes, and it gives me immense joy to see how refreshed you become from the tales I am able to tell. But you listen so badly! And that makes difficulties for me!"

As I said, she is a straightforward person who says whatever is lying heavily on her heart.

*Capesius:* Really? But I listen with all my comprehension.
*Felicia:* That's just it! You don't have the kind of comprehension that you ought to listen with.
*Capesius:* Really! Then what is lacking in my way of listening?
*Felicia:* I'm afraid you won't understand if I tell you!
*Capesius:* But I would like to understand.
*Felicia:* Well, if you listened properly, your etheric body would dance. And it doesn't dance.
*Capesius:* Why should my etheric body dance? How can I make it dance?
*Felicia:* Ah! First you must understand how the fairy tales actually come to me.

---

*At an afternoon gathering on the occasion of the first showing of eurythmy.
**See Rudolf Steiner, *Four Mystery Dramas*, especially *The Portal of Initiation*. Steiner Book Centre, Vancouver, Canada, 1973.

17

Now the good professor was a bit puzzled. He said: "You've told me so often that you receive the stories from the spiritual world, but—I'm really afraid to put it into words—it is beyond my comprehension why the beings who appear to you are always able to speak in the particular language of the persons who are listening to them and who later retell the story."

*Felicia:* Oh, that's just the point! That's just where your thoughts aren't clever enough. The beings don't tell me a story in words, they tell it in movements, and one has to understand what all their movements mean.

*Capesius:* How can I?

*Felicia:* Well, you learn how to let your heart go up into your head for a little while. Then you find that you have a special feeling for the motions the elves make, and the fairies, and the fairy princes. Then all those feelings stream into your larynx and you can tell a story. And if someone is listening properly, his etheric body will be dancing to it. But since you are unable to listen properly, you do not understand everything and much that I tell you is lost.

Now, we have caught up these words of Dame Balde to Capesius and have tried at least to organize the movements she described, the dances of the elves and gnomes, even of the angels, into a kind of movement system, a kind of movement language.

From many conversations with Felicia, it has come to light in a wonderful way that this subtle language can be made into something one can dance. One can even use the phrase, this "expression-language." And, to be brief, an "expression-dancing" is seen to be possible, an art of move-

18

ment, so to speak, which we have allowed ourselves to call the art of eurythmy: a kind of speech through movement, speech that can relate in a certain quite beautiful way to happenings in the spiritual world. For when Felicia let her heart radiate into her brain, she could actually, even though unconsciously, from her place in the world of forms, the world of the physical plane, catch glimpses of the world of the spirits of movement, and there she discovered her fairy tales.

How fine it would be, dear friends, if one could bring the kind of understanding that Capesius lacked to messages such as Felicia was able to bring from the spiritual world, if one could maintain complete quiet of the physical body and let one's etheric body dance! For this, we must first begin to find our way among a variety of movements that have a certain harmonious relation to movements that express cosmic tones and the cosmic word. What one was able to learn in the meetings with Dame Felicia will now become the foundation for our art of eurythmy. A beginning is now to be made with an art that stands on a boundary line, and for this reason it is important. In dance, if I may so express it, one can have the commonest, the most earthy impulse that lies nearest to human instincts and passions; yet, one can also embody the Dionysian element in the evolution of mankind!

A few eurythmy numbers will be presented to you. You will become familiar with the movements themselves. You will discover how human words and thoughts can be translated into these movements, and you will gradually learn how to "listen" to what is expressed in this new language.

But I beg you to remember in all this that we are involved in something that is at its very beginning.* You will be aware first of all, I hope, of the will initiative that stands

---

*Rudolf Steiner gave the first indications for eurythmy in 1912.

behind it, out of which, we believe, far more significant things can develop in the course of time than are yet there. You must also realize that a threefold intention lies behind eurythmy.

First, there must be an *esthetic* element. One could call it the element of beauty. Beauty is an immediate reflection of what goes on in the higher worlds in the form of movement. Thus, movements taken from the higher worlds and intensified are the artistic element.

But with this, a second element must at once be connected: the *pedagogical* element. The human soul will attain an unfoldment in its relation to the body that, in its connection to the soul worlds to which it belongs, corresponds to the vowel and consonant elements that stream through the world as cosmic word. In eurythmy these vowel and consonant elements are transformed into visible movements of the physical body. Thereby, if our beginnings will someday have achieved greater perfection, something quite different will have been accomplished than is achieved by the ordinary gymnastics and similar activities practiced at the present time, which are built only on physiological laws.

The third element is the *hygienic*. The fact that the human body will be adapted to a world of movement, also the idea of healthy human energy that will be infused into education, will further the development of the human organism and the human soul. Much that is unhygienic today in the outside world is caused by the fact that there is so little harmony between what the physical body has to do to adjust to the external world and what the etheric body, through its own inner mobility, demands from the physical body. This lack of coordination is what we would like to reduce by increasing the physical body's capacity for movement that corresponds to the needs of the etheric body.

And so it would be splendid if our young people—up to sixty or seventy years old—would acquire an understanding for this eurythmy that wants to bring the spiritual world down to the physical plane in ever more different ways. If our young people could gradually understand this art of expression, there would then be an increasing number of people among us to whom Dame Balde could say, "*Now* you don't listen so badly! You begin to understand me better!" She is a straightforward person and needs to judge us with her characteristic frankness so that we will respond earnestly. We must also learn to understand how she sees into the fairy tale world, and is then able to translate what she has seen into human words, because her heart is able to rise into her head.

# V

Please allow me to introduce our eurythmy program with a few words. I certainly do not want to "explain" the art forms we are attempting here, but to point to the sources of this new art.

As a matter of fact, eurythmy has been drawn forth from artistic foundations that are quite different from those of certain neighboring arts with which it could perhaps be easily confused. Eurythmy is a kind of silent speech. It is definitely not a system of haphazard gestures, nor has it anything to do with ordinary pantomime or the art of dance. It is opening up a fresh source for art through the fact that it uses the human being as the medium for its expression; that is, the human being with his inner inclinations to movement. The idea that underlies our endeavor comes altogether from what I would like to call Goetheanism, from Goethe's conception of art and his artistic perception. In this connection, however, one will have to accept various laws and facts that the people of today are not yet ready to acknowledge.

For instance, dear friends, everything connected with the human vocal organs (the larynx and neighboring parts) is in a remarkable way a miniature image of the entire structure of the human organism. In the larynx and its neighboring organs is to be found, formed of cartilage, the complete organic human structure. But the amazing thing about it is that the organs of the larynx do not continue inward and become muscular, as do other organs of movement, but

23

what rises out of the larynx as an impulse for movement goes out immediately into the surrounding air and sends forth tone or speech. Whoever has the faculty of sensible-supersensible observation (to use Goethe's expression), can study the movements the human larynx makes in order to send forth what becomes for us speech and song. These movements are completely unnoticed by us while we are listening to speech or song, but whoever does observe them can then transfer them to the entire human being.

For the sensible-supersensible observer this possibility of transference has a certain relation to the fact that an animal's vocal sounds reveal the character of its connection to surrounding nature and also to its own form. Whoever has intuitive perception will have no difficulty recognizing in the roar of a beast of prey a certain imitation of its form and, more particularly, of the movements coming from its muscular system. Similarly, he will recognize in a bird's song a wonderful expression of the bird's movement on the waves of the air and will observe that certain birds pour forth their particular pattern of song with certain definite accompanying movements.

To study such things carefully brings one to the moment when one is able to translate what normally remains invisible —the movements and inclinations to movement of the larynx and its adjacent organs—into visible movements of the entire human organism. One has then brought about a kind of silent speech, the instrument for it being the entire human being.

This, then, is what you will now see, with individual eurythmists making arm gestures as they move, or groups of eurythmists moving in space in definite relations to one another. In all that you see, there will be as little personal slant as you would find in a succession of tones forming a melody, or a structure of tones forming a chord. Eurythmy is in very truth a kind of music that is carried through space

24

by physical movements, and when two eurythmists, or two groups of eurythmists, present the same eurythmy number, there is no more personal aspect in the two presentations than when two pianists play the same sonata with their individual interpretations. Thus, any indulgence in play of gestures is here out of the question. Whatever personal expression you may see is due solely to the imperfecton that still clings to our eurythmic art.

Man, particularly man as he speaks, is really an expression of the entire universe. The fact, therefore, that here the entire human being becomes the medium for an art—usually, as you know, it is some musical instrument or other, but here it is the whole human being in movement—this fact fulfills what Goethe said so beautifully about man and his artistic activity: "Since man has been placed at the pinnacle of nature, he sees himself as a complete entity of nature that must now reach a similar height within himself. He now brings a new nature out of himself. He combines measure, order, harmony, significance, and finally rises to the production of a work of art." It is significant that he rises to this height when he uses his own organism as the means for his artistic expression.

Although eurythmy is still in its first stages, we believe that we have been able to achieve the beginning of a most important new art form. What is being attempted here now will have constant further development.

You will see this silent speech of eurythmy accompanied sometimes by music, sometimes by recitation. For what language expresses through the art of poetry can also be expressed by eurythmy in a completely parallel fashion. One must only understand that the movements meant for the air when the larynx makes them are in eurythmy given over to the muscles and, due to the fact that the entire human organism has now become the instrument for movement, these movements that normally happen in the larynx at tremendous speed are now made in eurythmy comparatively slowly.

In the recitation, too, you will find a rather different style from what is customary at the present time. Eurythmy wants to bring out of poetry its truly artistic content. It is good to remember how Goethe rehearsed his *Iphigenia* and his other verse-plays with the actors with a baton in his hand. Today people believe, but it is not true, that the essential task in recitation is to emphasize the prose content. In Goethe's time the more artistic natures—Schiller, Herder and others—all knew that beat, rhythm, in other words, the style underlying a poet's structuring of his language, is the real element in poetry, and that this must be our primary concern in recitation.

So we try here in our art of recitation to practice, I would like to say, an invisible eurythmy; that is, to handle our speech in such a way that what we do with our sounds and words parallels what you see the eurythmy doing on the stage.

You can see, I'm sure, that in our work here it is particularly the eurythmy that requires a return to certain fundamentals of art. These are the very fundamentals that today are practically ignored in artistic circles. Often today someone who considers himself to be exceedingly artistic is actually far from it for the reason that he is not putting the elements of true artistic style at the foundation of his work—elements of space, time, movement, for instance—but is bringing into the foreground, even in poetry, whatever constitutes a prose content. People get up to recite as if they wanted to impart a bit of prose information. They completely ignore the inner pulse of the poem.

So we believe that just by such performances as these, attention can be drawn in our time to true art.

In conclusion, dear friends, I would ask you to accept our program with good will. I feel I must say once more that eurythmy is in the first stages of its development. We are convinced that it will be carried forward by ourselves and by others from this simple beginning to ever greater perfection. It contains many varied possibilities for development, and will eventually take its place as a fully recognized art beside the older arts.

# VI

Before we show you our eurythmy, let me say a few words about it. It is not my intention to explain it. Artistic endeavors that need to be explained are not deserving of their name. Art speaks for itself. Even one's first impression of it should be intelligible. With eurythmy, however, we have undertaken to create an art from sources that are quite different from those previously known. Also, we are using a new artistic medium. Perhaps, therefore, you will allow me to speak briefly about these sources and this medium. The art of eurythmy is still only in its beginning, and only when it has become far more perfected will it be able to give what it is really intended to give.

You will see on the stage movements that individual eurythmists will make with their arms or with their whole body, and also movements of groups of eurythmists. None of this is pantomime or mime. Rather, the movements are based on a careful study of what happens in a human being when he is revealing the inner life of his soul through his speech. As with everything else that will go forth into the world from this Goetheanum, the art of eurythmy has also been created from Goetheanism, that is, from Goethe's conception of art and his artistic perceptions.

Goethe undertook to recognize the nature of a living being from its form. This may sound theoretical but it is truly not meant to be. More than is believed at the present time, men searching for knowledge will someday come back to Goethe's way of really penetrating to the nature of living things. First, however, certain prejudices that still exert a strong influence on present-day world conceptions have to be stripped away. In 1790 Goethe published a profound and supremely important essay, "An Attempt to Explain the Metamorphosis of Plants," that can point us in the right direction. Put briefly, Goethe proceeds to explain the form of the single leaf, whether simple or more complicated, as accounting for the *entire* plant, and the entire plant as being in its inner ideal nature only a complicated leaf. He regards the single plant, one might say, as a community of plants that appear as leaves that have undergone metamorphoses; petals, calyx, stamens, etc., are to him all metamorphoses of a leaf. This vivid conception of change from one kind of organ into another, this perception that the complicated structure of a complete living being has already been prepared in a certain sense in ideal form within its single organs: this, when it is developed further, is what will someday solve the mystery of organic life.

This conception of Goethe regarding the form of plants, which later he expanded to include animal forms, is here applied to the art of eurythmy but raised, of course, to an artistic level. Indeed, it is Goethe himself who builds the bridge from knowing to doing, to artistic activity. There is a beautiful saying of his that every artist should cherish: "He to whom Nature begins to reveal her open secrets, feels an irresistible longing for her most worthy representative, Art!" There Goethe relates artistic creation to true knowledge, knowledge that has nothing to do with theory but that belongs to immediate perception.

We are trying here to expand Goethe's ideas of form to human movement. We are making a careful study of the artistic movements that the larynx and its neighboring organs execute when someone speaks. It is not a question of those fine vibrations that are carried on the air from the speaker's larynx until they reach the listener's ear. Rather, it is the underlying inclinations to movement: the threads, as it were, on which those vibrations are strung. If one thinks of the long stem of a plant to which single tiny leaves are attached—like the locust, for instance—then one can imagine the tendencies that are present in the larynx and its neighboring organs, underlying the speech vibrations. These underlying impulses can be observed by—if I may use Goethe's expression—sensible-supersensible vision. Just as Goethe saw the whole plant as a single leaf whose form has become more and more complicated, so we are having the whole human being produce movements that otherwise are only produced in the region of the larynx and its neighboring organs. Thus we are transforming speech, of which the inclinations to movement are not noticed because ordinarily one is concerned only with its sound: we are transforming it into visible speech. Individuals or groups of individuals appear on the stage and make movements that normally are made only invisibly when one speaks. The sub-sensible impulse, I would like to call it, which underlies speech, is lifted out and revealed as movement by the entire human form or by groups of human beings.

In this connection I would like to point out from the sidelines, as it were, that through this work of ours it has been made possible to express many things that are felt strongly by contemporary artists. Today, numerous artists are creatively pursuing new forms of expression—impressionism, expressionism and various other styles. In impressionism the immediate impression has to be reproduced because men of the present day have lost the ability to penetrate to the inner nature of things as the great artists of earlier epochs could still do. So the impression is all there is left to hold on to. Expressionism, on the other hand, sets forth all that rises chaotically from the inner life, but in a way that more philosophical natures can hardly accept. All these ways are really only trying to answer in a new form

31

that old question of art: How does one manage to grasp artistic impressions without letting one's thoughts play a role?

Abstract thought will always kill real art. Art must be free to develop without it. We are able to keep it out of our eurythmy. This is not true of ordinary speech; that must serve the need for communication and it has already fallen too far into the conventions of practical life. The artist must seek satisfaction by reaching for what lies below speech, which is also, of course, an element of eurythmy.

In eurythmy we are able, apart from the conventional thought element that must be present in everyday speech, to eliminate thought entirely and to derive movement directly from the whole human being, from the human will. We have, therefore, an immediate experience for which the artistic medium is man himself, and in which the impression is of man himself. Since the human being is the medium, the instrument for this art, and since all affairs of the soul go immediately into movement, appealing directly to the senses, a unity of impressionism and expressionism is thereby brought about. Impressionism is there through the fact that it all speaks to the senses and to visual perception. Expressionism is there through the fact that it is the inner life of man that is being revealed by the eurythmy movements. All mime is excluded. An inner law underlies the movements that can be compared to the inner law relating melodic and harmonic elements in music.

So the recitation and the music that you will hear will also come to your vision as visible speech and visible music.

Those of you, dear friends, who have often been here before, will notice that we have been working recently to advance a little further, especially in the building up of the forms. Everything is, of course, still at an elementary stage but it is growing. We are our severest critics, and we know quite well how much of the detail is imperfect. We have still to bring the dramatic element into eurythmy; I have been

32

working toward this for some time, but the way to do it is not yet clear. The lyric and humorous elements have been highly successful in our recent performances. It is not merely the content of a poem but its actual structure—what the poet builds up out of its content—that we want to express in a new way through the dynamics of the eurythmy movements. That is our ideal. It is not the immediate feeling that should come to expression as in music, nor a trivial relation of inner soul experience and gesture, but something that has as lawful a structure as does speech itself.

Perhaps that gives you a little idea of what I wanted to say about the structure of eurythmy. You will find in it those truly artistic elements that otherwise have been completely lost today. Our time usually considers only the literal content of a poem, not the way the poem has been built up. Its meter, rhythm and structure are really the things that matter. We should remember that when Schiller was creating his most important poems he did not at first have the literal content of the poem in mind; there was just a kind of vague melody in his soul. This was the nucleus for his poem: he carried it as music strongly stirring within him. The words only came later. If someone is unable to appreciate this eurythmic element, he will also not understand what the really artistic element is in poetry. The recitation must bring out the really artistic element. It should not concentrate on the literal content with emphatic or muted voice and the like, even though this is nowadays the accepted ideal in the art of recitation. The truly important element to emphasize is the "how," the formative element, the arousal of thoughts and feelings quite apart from the literal content, which is only something to provide a base or to give direction to the artistic creation. It is not the artistic thing itself. If this were not so, one would simply not be able to have recitation accompanying eurythmy. Modern recitation as it is generally practiced is something that is no longer suitable to put by the side of eurythmy, which can be understood only as an *art*. When this comes about someday, it will be able to infuse a genuinely artistic element into its sister arts. Then there will be some prospect of this inartistic age coming once more into possession of true artistic feeling.

Eurythmy, this "visible speech," has also a therapeutic aspect, but lack of time prevents my speaking of this today. Also, its use in education is extremely important. Eurythmy is included in the curriculum of the Stuttgart Waldorf School as a prescribed subject. The good results derived from it can already be seen.

Dear friends, one is justified in a certain sense if one entertains a high regard for the gymnastics that have been developed in the modern age. Some individuals, however, who could see a little more deeply—Spengler, for instance—have held rather pronounced views against gymnastics. Anyone who does not succumb to modern prejudices will realize that gymnastics are derived from a purely physiological basis and therefore can only build up the physical body. That person will also realize that what a man needs most urgently today is initiative, soul initiative, will initiative. This can only be attained if "ensouled gymnastics"—namely, eurythmy—is introduced into education at the side of ordinary gymnastics. In eurythmy, in this "ensouled gymnastics," with every movement the child makes, not just his body but his whole being is brought into play. This must gradually be recognized because soul initiative, initiative of the will, must really be striven for as well as bodily development, which is the only part reached through gymnastics.

So today beside the artistic eurythmy there will be a few children's numbers. They are only to give an idea of how eurythmy can be taught to children as part of their school program.

For all of this, however, I hope I may still ask your indulgence. We ourselves—and this is meant quite seriously—are our severest critics of this beginning of artistic and pedagogical eurythmy. They will have to be developed much further, perhaps by others, because eurythmy is going to need a long period of time to evolve, such as the other arts have needed. Then—one who is deeply involved with eurythmy must hold this opinion—then eurythmy will be given a worthy place beside her older sisters, the arts with which humanity has long been blessed.

# VII

May I say a few words to introduce our eurythmy performance? Certainly not to explain it, because I am sure we agree that to explain a work of art is itself inartistic! Art must achieve its own effect through immediate perception. But eurythmy is an art form using a medium that today is still not well-known, and its creation springs from an artistic source that is likewise still unfamiliar. Perhaps, therefore, I may be permitted to say something about this artistic medium and its source.

Eurythmy can easily be confused with certain other related arts, which can here be fully acknowledged; there is nothing to be said against them. The simple fact is, however, that eurythmy is intended to be something else: not dance, not mime or pantomime or anything similar. It wants to use the artistic medium of actual visible speech. Those are not gestures in the ordinary sense that you will see on the stage, nor are they mime or pantomime; those limb movements and positions of the individual eurythmists or groups reveal real visible speech. You know, one can investigate what takes place supersensibly in a human being when he sings, when a singing tone comes forth from his bodily organism. One can also investigate what happens in a human being when speech sounds come forth from his organism. Through a kind of sensible-supersensible perception, one discovers at those moments that inclinations toward movement, movement-*intentions*—not the move-

37

ments themselves but the intentions-to-move—surge and weave through the entire human being.

These movement-intentions are checked at the moment of their origin and transformed into physical movements of single organs, the larynx and its neighboring organs, which are then given over to the air, thereby producing a tone, the singing tone of music or the sound of speech.

These movement-intentions that can be discovered in the human being by supersensible perception can be made manifest as a visible speech when they are taken over by the whole human being or groups of human beings. So those are the movements you will see in what are the most expressive limbs of the human organism, the arms and hands.

Now the single gesture should not be regarded as being already an expression of the soul, any more than should a single sound in speech be given a soul interpretation; the sound must be interpreted in its relation to other sounds. So also with eurythmy: it should make its immediate impression through its sequence of movements.

One can also make song visible when eurythmy is accompanied by music. When poems are recited, one brings them to visual perception through the visible speech of eurythmy. There is nothing fantastic about it; the movements come from the whole human organism with the same matter-of-factness as sound and tone come from the larynx.

One should therefore develop more interest in sequences of movements than in the separate movements. Music is not a matter of single isolated tones but of the melodic or harmonic progression of consecutive tones. Eurythmy is likewise not a matter of isolated gestures but of what is brought about creatively in a flow of movements.

Given this medium of visible song or speech, one has still to form it into something artistic. To begin with, eurythmy is bare speech, bare tone. The artistic activity only begins when one enters into a piece of music or a poem and becomes aware of the eurythmic element they contain hidden within them. For we must never forget that a true poet has this hidden eurythmy that is someday to become visible, already in his soul, even though unconsciously. If it is to be a real work of art, he fashions his poem out of his whole being, not from some single organ. That is why, when we present poems in eurythmy and accompany them with recitation and declamation, this must be of another kind than what is heard when just the prose content of a poem is communicated.

Poetry has to do with giving form to language. Whatever musical element there is in language, whatever imagery there is in the sounds, must be brought out by the recitation and declamation. Otherwise, it would be impossible to use them as accompaniments for the eurythmy. Emphasizing the prose content simply does not relate to what the eurythmy is doing. Actually, to develop the art of recitation and declamation as we want it, we have had to go back to earlier times that were more artistic than this present epoch, times when the musical element in language and its structure were considered more valuable than the prose content.

Now, precisely because the recitation and declamation must be of a different character, I am obliged to offer you an apology. Frau Dr. Steiner has asked me to apologize for the fact that although she is not an English woman, yet it is she who will recite the English poems. She is obliged to do so because it is important to have this new art of recitation and declamation, which is only at the beginning of its development, presented here. We must wait for it to grow fully in the various languages.

Beside the eurythmy that you will now see, there are two other forms of it that I will just mention. One is therapeutic eurythmy. All the movements that are used here on the stage in an artistic undertaking are taken from the human organism with just as much matter-of-factness, just as much necessity as speech itself. They represent the healthy human organism. Now, not these exact movements but others metamorphosed from them, constitute curative eurythmy. You can find curative eurythmy now being worked out in our medical institutes in Arlesheim and Stuttgart as a special therapeutic measure. One can already see how useful eurythmy is going to be in hygienic and therapeutic work when it is gradually given other forms than the purely artistic one that is being presented today.

The third sphere of eurythmy is the pedagogical. I won't go into that now because tomorrow we are going to have the pleasure of showing you some children's eurythmy, and I will introduce it then with a few words. The importance of pedagogical eurythmy has been apparent ever since the founding of the Waldorf School in Stuttgart, where eurythmy is included in addition to gymnastics as a prescribed subject. As naturally as children grow into speech and song, do they grow into this visible speech and visible song.

So I now have only to say what I must never neglect to mention: that we would ask you, dear friends, to be charitable! Eurythmy is still at the very beginning of its development and every art form at first must of necessity be imperfect. We are our severest critics; we know what our eurythmy still lacks, and we are trying—I would say, from month to month—to improve it.

For instance, today you will see something that only a year ago was missing. The entire stage picture has been made eurythmic; you will not only see the moving eurythmists, but you will also see lighting effects that correspond to the successive scenes of the eurythmy. There, likewise, the chief interest must not be accorded to single moments of color, but rather to the sequence—I would like to say, the "demonic " sequence—of the lighting effects, which should relate exactly to the sequence of the eurythmic picture.

While acknowledging the present immaturity of our eurythmy, and bearing in mind the artistic medium with which we are working and the artistic sources from which we are able continually to create, one might say that this art is capable of being perfected eventually to an immeasurable degree, since it uses an instrument that must be recognized as the greatest artistic tool—the human being himself, the entire organism of the human being. All cosmic secrets and laws are contained in him. If, therefore, one derives visible speech from the whole human being, one has found something that can truly reveal the totality of cosmic secrets and laws. Man is a microcosm, and if this microcosm is used as an artistic medium, it can lend expression to mysteries that pervade the entire cosmos. So one may expect that in spite of its present shortcomings eurythmy will in time to come be so perfected that finally it will stand as a fully recognized art form beside the older, more familiar forms.

And now a word about the performance. We have divided the program into two parts. At the end of the first part, a scene from one of my Mystery Plays will be presented. The play portrays the development of a man who gradually gains entrance into the supersensible world. It is especially appropriate to use eurythmy to show what connects man with the supersensible world.

The scene will show how everything that Johannes Thomasius has experienced with his friends Capesius, Strader and others, has so deepened in his soul that it appears to him in the form of his Double. His own youth appears before his inner sight and the Guardian of the Threshold appears, before whom a man stands when he enters the spiritual world. Johannes also sees another figure—Ahriman, the embodiment of slyness, of evil. These are inner happenings

41

in the soul of Johannes Thomasius. Whatever takes place in the supersensible sphere is presented by eurythmy and is recited by Frau Dr. Steiner. Johannes Thomasius is portrayed on the stage as an ordinary physical human being. Everything that is conceived of as physical must be shown on the stage also as physical, while everything that happens in the supersensible world can be presented on a higher level through eurythmy.

At the beginning of the second part of the program another scene from one of the Mystery Plays will be presented in which the luciferic powers of mysticism, of sentimentality, appear before Capesius, and also the ahrimanic powers of evil, cunning, cleverness, guile. Capesius does not appear because he is experiencing this happening as a dream. This is indicated by a special figure who speaks before Capesius comes to himself out of his dream vision. So we have scenes from the Mystery Dramas at the end of the first part of the program and the beginning of the second.* I trust this is clear.

---

*At the end of the first part of the program, Scene Four of *The Souls' Awakening* was presented, and after the intermission, part of Scene Six of *The Guardian of the Threshold*. The "special figure," a eurythmist, presented in eurythmy what in a dramatic performance of the play is spoken in chorus by Philia, Astrid and Luna: "Thoughts hovered near . . ."

# VIII

May I say a few words to introduce our modest euryth-my program? Certainly what is offered as art should not be explained; that would be an inartistic beginning! Art must achieve its own effect through immediate perception and this is especially true for eurythmy. Since eurythmy, how-ever, is emerging as a new art, created from new artistic sources that today are still unfamiliar, and since it uses an artistic medium that is also still unfamiliar, perhaps I may speak briefly about these things.

What you are now going to see on the stage is definitely not to be looked upon as dancing, or as mime or panto-mime. It is visible speech. One can actually observe by sensible-supersensible perception, if I may use Goethe's ex-pression, that when a person sings or speaks, his entire organism seeks only special, concentrated expression through his larynx and its neighboring organs. Singing, that is, the music that comes from the human being, and also speech, are of such a nature that they engage his entire being. Something that is happening in all the rest of his organism is only just indicated by his speech and is metamorphosed in a special way in his specific organs for singing and speaking.

One can actually observe what lies behind human speech. One sees inclinations toward movement, inclina-tions toward form. Now, one can carry these over to the whole human being—suitably changed so that they can be *seen*— while we do not see the movements of the special speech organs but *hear* them as they are transformed into

43

the movements of the air. What normally is heard in song or speech is seen in the eurythmy movements. For this reason, a eurythmy gesture is something quite different from a dance gesture or from a gesture in mime or pantomime. Just as little as one can use any haphazard speech sound to express a particular soul experience, just so little can one use any random eurythmy gesture to express it. For a human being to express himself clearly through eurythmy, there are definite movements to be used in relation to definite sounds, definite word stresses, word formations, etc. Also, therefore, one should not expect to devote one's perception to the single gestures, but just as when hearing a melody one listens to the succession of tones, so here one should be watching a flow of movements—whether a single eurythmist is creating the flow or groups of eurythmists are moving in eurythmy forms.

Eurythmy can indeed be thought of as moving sculpture. Someone who has a feeling for such things could say that when we stand before a statue in its stillness, we have there a vivid portrayal of human silence, soul silence. In contrast, what is expressed here when the human being is in movement, is the human soul when it is stirred. Gestures are used that belong as specifically to human soul experiences as speech sounds belong to them. Thus, perhaps this new art could be described as sculpture-in-movement.

We want to find the way gradually to assemble the entire stage scene so that it will be a unified expression of eurythmy. Those of you who have been here often will notice, I'm sure, how we have worked in these last months to improve the stage lighting, not by simply adding light sequences, but by learning to create color sequences that relate precisely to the eurythmy they are accompanying. Here, too, one should not focus one's attention upon single momentary effects, but rather upon the progression of the lighting from one eurythmy movement to the next, or perhaps upon the re-

44

straint that the lighting exerts as it accompanies the single eurythmy numbers.

Eurythmy can also point the way back to a more artistic comprehension of recitation and declamation than is to be found today in this rather inartistic age. Apart from a few individuals who do realize that something different must be striven for, people today still recite and declaim in such a way that only the prose content of a poem is brought to expression. They say they emphasize the prose in this way or that as the depth of their feelings dictates. But a real poet does not at first trouble his soul with the prose content at all; he is pursuing an elusive melody, or some harmonious musical element, or he is working with the structure of the language. A real poet—if he is an artist—before attending to the prose content of his poem, must be listening to an inner necessity, something that is weaving, something quite alive, rounding itself out and rounding itself off, perhaps plunging deeper or reaching higher to another level where he will finally be able to gather up what has been forming and give it words in this or that thought. The truly artistic form has at first nothing to do with the prose thought that is to be expressed, for instance, in an octet of two four-line strophes and a sextet of two three-line strophes. It has only to do, so to speak, with initiating a going-forward and a return in the first two octet strophes, and in the last two sextet strophes with a contemplation of what went forward and a glancing back at the return. This is the kind of shaping and forming in which one lives when one is creating a sonnet—the Italian sonnet—out of truly artistic feeling, artistic fantasy.

So it is that something always lies underneath, as with Schiller, for instance, who in his greatest lyric poetry never concerned himself at first with the prose content, but only strung it on afterward when he had finally found the thread of a melody running vaguely within him. With Goethe it was more an indistinct feeling. Goethe lived more in indis-

45

tinct feelings than Schiller. Such things must definitely come to expression in the recitation and declamation that accompanies eurythmy. One simply cannot declaim or recite in a prosy way when one accompanies eurythmy!

There will also be visible song in the program, where the eurythmy accompanies music played by single instruments or by an ensemble. We have undertaken to perform both for you, eurythmy with music and eurythmy with recitation. When one recites for eurythmy, one must pay attention to the structure of the language and to the musical element. In this sense, the art of recitation and declamation must return to what it was in more artistic centuries than the present one. What we are trying to develop here into a real art can today still be regarded as strange. When someday our age returns to a really artistic level, it will be understood.

But I must say, as always, that we ourselves are our severest critics; we well know what has still to be perfected, and we beg our audience to be charitable! Eurythmy is only in its infancy, but we know how immeasurable can be its development.

I would like now to mention that in the second part of the program we will present a scene from Part II of Goethe's *Faust*, where the Four Grey Women and particularly Worry (*Sorge*) are on the stage. It must be said that the style of eurythmy is on a higher level than that to which the stage is accustomed; every eurythmy gesture, every eurythmy movement must be lifted to a higher level of artistic style because it springs from the entire human organism. Therefore, eurythmy is especially suited to portray something in drama—not in lyric poetry—something in drama that reaches into the supersensible world. There are many scenes in Goethe's *Faust* where the human soul enters into relation with the supersensible, as in this one where the Four Grey Women appear. Faust must, of course, be portrayed as a physical man by the usual naturalistic stage art. But what

46

goes on in his soul, what he beholds through his relation to the supersensible world, what attains through Goethe to dramatic representation in the Four Grey Women (for it is not mere allegory): this can be translated especially well into eurythmic language.

So the ordinary stage style and the eurythmy style will be combined. Perhaps you will see that certain parts of *Faust*, certain scenes, especially in Part II, with their more special language, gain their proper significance on the stage when they are presented not naturalistically but on a higher artistic level through eurythmy.

There are two other sides to eurythmy. One is curative eurythmy, in which the movements that you are now going to see made artistically are transformed. All eurythmy flows out of the healthy human organism, bringing it into movement such as a healthy organism demands. The eurythmy movements can also, therefore, be used therapeutically, as is already to be seen in our Arlesheim clinic and elsewhere.

A third element is pedagogical eurythmy. A school curriculum can include eurythmy by the side of gymnastics as, one might say, an ensouled gymnastics. In the Stuttgart Waldorf School we are already convinced that from the youngest child to the oldest, the eurythmy works strongly on the will in such a way that the children find their way into eurythmic speech as easily as they are used to finding their way into ordinary speech. Particularly in the "ensouled gymnastics" one can see what an important element eurythmy is for education. One sees a child's body, soul and spirit all growing healthy through its use. In eurythmy, the living human being is used as medium. Goethe said that man finds himself confronted by nature and takes measure, harmony, order, significance from it, rising by use of them to the creation of a work of art. So it may well be said that man, as a microcosm, holds all the secrets of the world within himself. If, therefore, these secrets are discovered and lifted into

47

view through the art of eurythmy, then, because man himself is the instrument, and nothing external, the secrets of the human form can be revealed through him. Man can be a reflection of the secrets of the larger world, of the entire macrocosm.

For the very reason that eurythmy lifts harmony, order, measure, significance out of man and reveals them through him, one can say that while eurythmy is today still in its beginning, it will undoubtedly go through a broad development and someday be able to take its place as a fully recognized, valuable art among the older arts.

# IX

It is my pleasant task to introduce our eurythmy performance but forgive me for not speaking in the language of this country. I hope you will excuse my inability and allow me to use the language to which I am accustomed.

The eurythmy you are going to see will be performed by individuals and groups. The movements they will be making are not gestures in the usual sense of the word, nor are they pantomime or mime or any other art of movement. They are movements presenting actual visible speech. I say this not to explain the artistic content of the performance. Art must speak for itself through its immediate impact; any explanation of a work of art is itself inartistic! Our eurythmy, however, springs from artistic sources that today are still unfamiliar, and it uses an artistic form that likewise is unfamiliar. Perhaps, therefore, you will allow me to say a few words about them.

In ordinary human speech and song we have to do with something that has evolved quite consistently according to certain laws out of the human organs for speech and song. We have the human will coming forth from the deepest core of the human being, and also thought that is poured out of the nervous system in a most complicated way into the speech organs. These two elements flow together in speech, and a third element, feeling, unites what thought on the one side and will on the other want to bring to expression.

Now, it is really the thought element in speech that produces most obstacles for the poet, the real poet. Thoughts

49

are an inartistic element. But thought can be studied, and everything you are now going to see of the eurythmic art of movement is based entirely upon careful study by—if I may use Goethe's expression—sensible-supersensible perception. One can observe, for instance, the movements that the larynx and its neighboring organs are making at the moment when a word or a singing tone is being given over to the air. One comes gradually to the discovery that even ordinary speech actually comes about by virtue of a transformation of gestures—not the everyday gestures by which we normally accompany our conversation, but gestures that live within us while we are speaking and that do not come to external, physical view at all. The human brain is such a complicated organ that it is extremely difficult to see what happens when someone speaks or sings. Actually, for every vowel, for every consonant, a specific gesture is produced, but is held back and transformed. Through a complicated expedient of the nervous system, each specific gesture is made into a picture, and an after-image of the gesture is, so to say, entrusted to the vibrating air that in speaking or singing streams out from the human organism. It is just this—the gesture that is held back when one speaks or sings and then by a mysterious human power is committed to the air stream —it is just this that is brought out and revealed by the art of eurythmy. Every vowel, every consonant, the complete structure of a word, of a sentence will now appear before you in the movements made by individual eurythmists and groups of eurythmists on the stage.

It is especially the arms and hands, the most expressive part of the human body, that speak to you in this visible speech. One should not, however, try to link single gestures that the eurythmist makes to single words, to the soul content of single words. In music, for instance, one listens for the way the tones follow one another to form a melody; so also in eurythmy one looks for a sequence of movements. One could really say that we are talking about a melody of movements. One is not expected to interpret single gestures; rather, a sweep of movement should have the power, at the moment that it is being seen and artistically enjoyed, to evoke the impression, the mood, that the poet or composer wanted to create.

For some time, we have been working to make the entire stage picture relate to the eurythmy as it is being performed on the stage. We have tried to develop the stage lighting so that the entire stage picture is, as it were, an extension of the eurythmy itself. Thus, it is not a matter of single moments of separate lighting effects, but of an harmonious, melody-like sequence of lighting.

So eurythmy can accompany a piece of music with visible song, singing visibly as one would sing with tones, and it can make visible what the poet has expressed in artistic language.

It is of the greatest importance that when eurythmy is accompanying a poem, the recitation and declamation shall also express what is being expressed in the visible speech, the eurythmy. In the work of a true poet—in the structure of his language, the way he forms his sentences, the way he uses meters and all the artistic elements of language—there already lies a hidden eurythmy. Since here our recitation and declamation will always parallel the poetic content of the eurythmy, you will realize that we lay less value on the literal prose content of a poem than on the true artistry of the language, the melodic quality, the imaginative, pictorial element that a real poet has put into his work. Some coming epoch more artistic than this one will, among other things, return to the fine art of recitation and declamation, and will emphasize the musical, sculptural, colorful elements in poetry instead of pointing up its prose content as is generally done today. Here, the recitation and declamation must sound forth in harmony, in parallel mood, with what happens visibly on the stage.

So, my dear friends, one achieves a higher degree of style than is possible with the ordinary art of mime. Particularly today you will realize this is so because you are going to see eurythmy and acting on the stage at the same time, in a scene from the second part of *Faust:* "Worry (*Sorge*) and the Four Grey Women." You will see Faust presented quite naturally, as a man is usually portrayed expressing his normal soul life. That can be presented by ordinary acting. But then Faust is confronted by the Four Grey Women and Worry, who are really the embodiment of supersensible powers, supersensible forces. These are made physically perceptible and thereby is shown the relation an individual human soul can have to the supersensible, spiritual world. In such an instance, where something spiritually perceptible, spiritually experienced is to be put on the stage—something not physical, not earthly—there eurythmy can be especially useful. In this *Faust* scene that we are showing today, you will see Faust presented in the usual style of the stage. What the Four Grey Women and particularly Worry bring to Faust, however, you will see presented by eurythmy accompanied by recitation just for the eurythmy.

We can say, therefore, that particularly when a more subtle style is needed for something on the stage that goes beyond the usual naturalism, the art of eurythmy can be experienced in its true character.

Today as always I must beg you to be charitable! We are our severest critics and we know that our eurythmy is only at the very beginning of its development. It will be much further perfected. While we ourselves are only involved in its beginning, we know how immeasurable is the possibility of its development because it has, not the external instruments, but the human being for its artistic medium. In the human being all the secrets, all the laws of the cosmos are assembled. He is a microcosm. By revealing him through the visible speech of eurythmy, by drawing forth from him what moves the soul, what awakens the human spirit, one really draws from the whole human being all cosmic secrets in miniature. Goethe said about art, "Since man stands at nature's pinnacle, he sees himself as a complete nature that must again climb to a pinnacle. He strives toward the height by permeating himself with all perfections and virtues, by calling forth choice, order, harmony, significance, and finally rises to the creation of works of art."

Likewise, one can say that in eurythmy not only are order, harmony, measure, significance taken from the surrounding world but out of man himself because all world secrets are contained in him as in a microcosm. The cosmos can tell us its most intimate secrets through these human movements; through them the soul can most purely, most profoundly, most intimately reveal itself. For the very reason that eurythmy uses the human being for its medium, one can hope that although today it is still rather unusual, it will in the coming years arouse more and more interest, and also will be more and more perfected as it develops, so that one day it will be given a place beside the older sister arts as a fully acknowledged young art in its own right.

# X*

We are now going to present a short program of eurythmy. This new art must be distinguished from the art of mime and from the art of the dance. Certainly we would not raise the slightest objection to those arts. But, to put it simply, eurythmy is intended to be something entirely different. In mime one makes gestures to indicate something, to call attention to something, while in dance one uses exaggerated gestures in which the soul loses itself. Eurythmy uses gestures, too, and movements of the body, but they are neither for indicating nor for exaggerating. Perhaps one could call the eurythmy gestures expressive, in the sense that words are expressive, that everything coming from a human being by way of his speech is expressive.

Speech, too, has to do essentially with a kind of art of gesture, but the gesture is made within the person who speaks and is carried in the stream of air coming from his larynx. This outcoming air stream takes on the exact forms of the words and sentences. Were one to see it, one would see that this is so. In the stream of air, the speaker's will and thinking are flowing together out of his soul. Will is the element that in a certain sense gives the air a radial direction, while thought cuts across the air waves in some rhythm or other. In a poet's artistic shaping of the language to create a poem, we see him striving as far as possible to conquer the thought element that predominates in prose. Already in the

*During the pedagogical course at the Goetheanum. GA 306

art of rhetoric—speaking that aims to use beautifully flowing speech—the intention is to give a form to the language itself. A poet's chief endeavor is to overcome the purely prosaic thought element by making every possible use of musical, sculptural, colorful elements of language, to express what wants to be brought to expression by the very shape he gives the language.

When, therefore, it comes to reciting the poem, a real art of recitation and declamation—something that is certainly not being cultivated in today's inartistic world—a real art of recitation and declamation has the corresponding task of voicing the words musically, sculpturally, colorfully. If, for instance, a poem describes the passion that is moving a soul, this will have to be expressed in the recitation by a different rhythm in the flow of words from a rhythm that, for instance, would express sorrow or withdrawal into the soul.

Prose is nowadays of such a nature that it describes the full range of a soul experience simply and completely by the meaning of its words, without concern for any other element of language. In poetry, by contrast, one endeavors to bring the language into play so as to reveal by various artistic means what otherwise is only to be found in the word content. It is therefore not real recitation and declamation when one emphasizes the prose content of a poem as is usually done today. Recitation or declamation should mean that the speaker takes pains to bring out that hidden eurythmy that the poet has put into his language. If one is aware of the musical element and the sculptural and colorful elements in speech, if one realizes that these elements can be revealed not only by dance movements but also by something else, by certain expressive gestures that are to be found in the human bodily organism, then one has reached the possibility of creating an actual visible speech. This visible speech can already be seen in the gestures made, say, by a rather temperamental person who feels he cannot express what he wants to express just through the sounds of speech and so he helps his speech along by making gestures. But these, one might say, are babbling gestures. As a small child starts to speak by babbling and then advances to articulate speech, so the ordinary gestures one makes while speaking are related to the eurythmy gestures you are now going to see on the stage. Eurythmy has indeed come about in this way: that by sensible-supersensible vision one has been able to observe the forms that are created by the air streaming out from the larynx and its neighboring speech organs during speaking and singing.

Now one lets these forms flow into the air in the way they usually do in speaking or singing, but shaped now by visible human hands and arms. Those are the most expressive human limbs; the rest of the body can also make eurythmy movements but with less character. The forms correspond to soul experiences; they must flow into the air so clearly that what they are expressing can be immediately experienced. So when something is played or recited, one hears the artist's composition of tones or of words and at the same time one sees with one's eyes the eurythmy that had lain hidden in the music or poem, and that is now being revealed in visible song or visible speech. That, then, is eurythmy: an individual in movement, or a group of individuals in movement, or several groups relating to one another, all portraying the human soul by translating speech or song into movement.

So eurythmy is not an invention of chance gestures to add to a poem or a piece of music. Just as one cannot embody what one wants to say with words in any random collection of speech sounds, for the reason that every single state of soul has definite sounds corresponding to it, so also a soul experience cannot be expressed by some random gesture suddenly invented, for the reason that every soul experience has a definite gesture corresponding to it. So when you find a series of vowels in a poem, you can be sure that the poet has used it to express something musically, colorfully; naturally, you must take care of that in your recitation. You cannot express the poem with certain sounds one day, other sounds another, because the sounds relate to harmonies existing between physical organism and soul life. In precisely the same way, there are only definite movements to be made in eurythmy. For a certain motif you will always see the same gesture. Yes, down to the smallest vowel or consonant, everything has its own fixed gesture. In speech, E is a quite distinct sound; in eurythmy, too, it is a quite distinct gesture. But then, just as in reciting poetry an E can be spoken brightly or dully, loudly or softly, long or short, so also in eurythmy the specific gesture for E can be made in various ways.

So you can see that in eurythmy it is of prime importance that when a gesture is being shaped, it shall be shaped really artistically. Every movement must be formed artistically. Then something will have been created that is a truly independent art able to take its place beside the other arts, an art of movement in space.

Of course, eurythmy is today only at the beginning of its development. But it holds promise of many, many phases of growth because it is making use of what one would say is the most perfect human instrument, the human body itself. The human organism contains all cosmic secrets and all cosmic laws; it is a microcosm confronting the macrocosm. Eurythmy makes more perfect use of this microcosm, the human body, than does the art of mime with its indicating gestures. These are only guessed at, so to say, and thereby an intellectual element is allowed to enter. Eurythmy also makes more perfect use of the whole bodily organism than does the art of the dance, which overflows in its movement into space. Eurythmy can also overflow in its movements, but it should not do so in such a way that it gushes, as it were, in the movement; its movement should always be held in control by the inner laws of the human organism. In eurythmy there can be no movement that does not show by its very nature that an element of soul lies behind it.

If, indeed, eurythmy is occasionally called upon to express something similar, may I say, to what we in our everyday speech stoop to express by mimicking facial expressions —for instance, smirking to show that we consider ourselves above something or other, drawing the corners of our mouth down to mock at someone, and so forth—thus, when we express certain earthy feelings by mimicking: well, eurythmy can stoop to mimicking, too—*if the poet wants that*. But if from its own impulse eurythmy falls into mimicry, then it has become impure.

Similarly, eurythmy can fall into dancing when, for example, it has to express that someone is hitting another, or that someone is rushing about in a passion. But this overflowing, this exaggeration must be kept within eurythmy itself, for when eurythmy becomes dance, it is vulgar.

Eurythmy must stay clear of these two precipices, mime and dance. It must regard them as strict boundaries; otherwise, it will fall into impurity or vulgarity.

Obviously, then, eurythmy must be recognized as a distinct and separate art. This is easiest to see when one is looking at tone eurythmy. The eurythmist is not dancing to the music, she is singing to it, singing-with-movements. If someone would once experience the difference between dancing to orchestra music and "singing" to it (singing-with-movements), he would then have the right feeling for the place eurythmy holds between the art of mime and the art of the dance.

Eurythmy uses the human body more perfectly than

59

either of these two arts, and one may hope, since the human body is the most perfect instrument, that eurythmy itself will be able to become more and more perfected.

Let me add something else. We have been trying recently to perfect our coordination of stage lighting and eurythmy in order to have a more perfect stage picture.

So one may hope that eurythmy will someday be ready to take its place as a fully recognized art by the side of the other arts. I have tried to show that it has not been formed from any of them; it is and will be a distinct art next to the others, an art that draws its substance from artistic sources perhaps still unfamiliar, and that uses an artistic language that is also perhaps unfamiliar.

# XI

Goethe speaks of sensible-supersensible perception as enabling one to grasp something artistically. If one tries to grasp artistically the human speech and song system, to grasp it in its broadest aspect, one discovers something that lies behind speech and behind song; one finds something that has to do with the whole human being, in contrast to the fact that speech and song as such have only to do with a single small group of physical organs. Who does not feel that whenever he gives himself to speech or song, his whole soul is participating—indeed, so much so that he feels his soul weaving and pulsing through his whole organism? One can even say, at least when our speech is not merely serving to impart some conventional information or purely logical sequence of thought, but when it is shaped artistically, that then the entire human being wants to be expressed, and this expression, this revelation of the whole human being is merely concentrated in a limited group of speech organs.

One could ask what movement has to take place within us when we sing something or say something. One does discover certain movements that are actually transformed by the speech organs, the larynx and its adjoining organs, into air movements and are in this way thrown out, as it were, to the outside world. One discovers that these movements can also be traced in reverse, traced back to where they originate in the human being. Ordinarily, one finds that they have been suppressed. A man responds to everything he hears said to him by these inner movements, or he suppresses them; one then finds them replaced by the sympathy he feels toward the world and his fellowmen as he listens to what is spoken.

Similarly, when we speak ourselves, there is the unconscious desire to accompany what we say by these movements, these gestures, but we suppress them because what we want to say finds its expression through the sounds of speech.

But everyone knows that in song and also in speech that is formed artistically there is something one calls style, that language is shaped in a certain way, given a certain style by a poet. He brings in a rhythmic element, he makes use of certain meters, he introduces word motifs like melodies into his language, he responds to a certain fantasy in his use of speech sounds.

All this is something that lies at the foundation of speech but does not enter permanently into it. Someone who has an intimate feeling for human life can sense that when he gives over to his larynx what is in his soul, he really externalizes it. I would like to say that he gives it over to the objective-spiritual sphere of life.

Now, what the soul experiences more inwardly can be brought to expression through "stylized" gestures, and it is eurythmy that thus brings it to expression so that there comes about an actual visible speech and an actual visible song. The entire content of eurythmy, all the gestures of individual eurythmists or of groups of eurythmists, are taken from the human organism as precisely, as properly as are the speech sounds themselves, that is, the vowels, consonants, sentence structure, and so forth.

The visible speech and visible song that arise in this way can be quite correctly understood if one follows how the recitation and declamation, and also the musical numbers, are accompanied here by eurythmy movements. At first, people are inclined to regard the tone eurythmy as dance, but eurythmy is not dance. It is really singing-in-movement, in which the singing is not done by tone but by movement. One only begins to understand eurythmy properly when one is able to regard it, not as dance, but as moving song, song-in-movement.

In the same way, the eurythmy movements accompany what is being expressed by the speech sounds. In the speech of civilized peoples today there lives a spiritual element, an objective element, that becomes more and more separated from the individuals themselves. One feels, and quite rightly, an unpleasant quality in the more sophisticated modern languages when a subjective element enters the speech: when something is over-emphasized, or when the prose content is stressed, and the like. One feels it is almost lewd when too much of a subjective element is brought in. Speech should spiritualize the soul element and thereby detach it more or less from the speaker. We can take what comes to expression in "stylized" speech and put it back into human movement. Then the soul element is revealed in the moving human being; his movements—especially those of the most expressive part of his body, his hands and arms —become a visible speech. When we give voice to consonants, the happenings in the outside world are expressed by them rather objectively. When we speak the vowels, there live in them the feelings that we entertain toward these happenings, but separated from us, spiritualized. I would like to say that with the visible speech of eurythmy—if, for instance, a poem is presented—one lives in it entirely as soul. What lives in one's spirit is ensouled by eurythmy.

Eurythmy is able to translate the vowel sounds as well as the consonant sounds into movements. When the vowels are formed into eurythmy movements, they reveal what the soul experiences in its deepest inwardness. With the consonants, it is man's lively relation to all things that the eurythmy brings to expression.

63

While our ordinary speech tends more and more to spiritualize our soul experiences, eurythmy, by its very nature, stresses the soul quality of our inner experiences. Indeed, every movement made here on the stage is a visible expression of the most intimate soul experience.

When, therefore, we accompany eurythmy by recitation and declamation, that "hidden eurythmy" that the poet weaves invisibly into his poem must also be given expression. We cannot recite and declaim as is usually done, where the really artistic elements of language are not considered at all but only the prose content is emphasized.

Here we want to recite and declaim in such a way that the artistic elements of the language will be brought into prominence. The tone structure and tone quality of the recitation must coincide with the eurythmy movements. When the recitation or declamation is intoned and the eurythmy movements made simultaneously as if together they were an orchestral ensemble, then it is as if the speech sounds themselves were part of the style that the poet is creating, and as if they were able to make the style more human. The style of a poem is the element that raises it to a supersensible level, while the speech sounds themselves bring the supersensible realm down to our human level of experience.

When we are watching eurythmy and listening to the recitation and declamation, the eurythmy continually raises the recitation and declamation to "style" before our eyes. One has the feeling, therefore, that in performing eurythmy we must enter as far as possible into the poet's style. It must parallel our endeavor to bring recitation and declamation back to those earlier times when Goethe rehearsed his iambic dramas with the actors with a baton in hand like a choral director, showing that he valued an artistic treatment of his language far more than emphasis of the prose content. We, too, must return to the secrets of imaginative and musical speech formation if we would raise recitation and declamation to an art. At the same time we will be developing a truly artistic support for the eurythmy.

But there is also the need to support the style of our eurythmy in other areas. Those of you, dear friends, who have come often to the eurythmy performances here, will have noticed our efforts lately to add new lighting effects to the stage scene. These are not intended to apply to single gestures in a naturalistic way, but just as in music a melody is only to be found in a series of tones, so here in the eurythmy lighting what we are trying to achieve should be looked for in the lighting sequences. We want to place the moving eurythmy picture within sequences of lighting that relate and belong to it, sequences that then are themselves a kind of "light eurythmy."

Today, as always before our programs, I must ask you to remember that we are only at the beginning of this art of eurythmy. We know better than anyone else our imperfections. What eurythmy is intended to be will only be fully realized in the future. Eurythmy makes much more perfect use of a human being in motion than does the art of mime, for instance. Mime uses the moving human being for, so to say, accompaniment. Eurthymy requires that everything within man shall be, I would like to say, brought out so that he is like a living, visibly active larynx. It tries in its movements to present artistically everything that lies hidden within the human form.

If one thinks of man as a microcosm that contains a whole world within himself, then one can say that eurythmy has a future, because it is through eurythmy that the most important, the most profound world secrets will come to be revealed artistically. If man is a microcosm and contains all world secrets within himself, these will become manifest to

65

the eye. Then one can use the entire man as a medium of expression. That is what eurythmy wants to do. So one may allow oneself to hope that although eurythmy is a young art, it will nevertheless gradually develop to such perfection that it will finally be able to take its place in full recognition beside the older accepted arts.

# XII

From various comments that have been made recently concerning the eurythmy performances, one realizes what a long time it takes for people to reach an artistic understanding of what eurythmy is meant to be. One notices that ordinary people who simply give themselves up to an artistic pleasure let the eurythmy affect them through their immediate perception, and indeed out of their ingenuousness soon gain an understanding for it. But people who are accustomed to pondering for long periods over art, people who, for instance, write critiques on art, have great difficulty in accepting eurythmy from a genuinely artistic point of view. They often say that there is too much intellectual content to eurythmy; it is extraordinarily clever—this is the latest comment heard—but there is so much intellectuality in those movements!

Actually, as a matter of fact, there is not the slightest particle of intellectual content in them! That's the amazing fact about eurythmy, that it contains nothing intellectual at all, and you understand it best if you don't pile up a stack of thoughts about it but simply open your artistic eye to it. For eurythmy is really just to look at and accept in an immediate visible impression. It is to take in as simply as one takes in speech. With speech one simply lets it come to one. One learns it so early in one's childhood that it is just there without question. It has been pushed up out of the unconscious; it is not formed by intellectual forces. It would be sad indeed if the forming and pronouncing of words and learning their meanings had to be thought through by a child before he spoke. If that were so, a child would never learn to speak. Fortunately, one does not learn speech. A child experiences it while imitating it, just as he grows. The child does not draw his growth out of thoughts but simply responds to his human nature and grows. So it is also with speech; a child does not learn it in successive details but it grows through his living together with his surroundings.

Perhaps it looks as though there must surely be something more underlying eurythmy than underlies what we call learning to speak. But really, there is nothing else at all. With eurythmy one has to do with a genuine visible speech that is drawn from the human being in just as matter-of-fact a way as ordinary speech is drawn out of him. Actually, a person does something similar to gesturing whenever he speaks, but he is not aware of it; he does not notice that he is sending gusts of air out on his breath continually like gestures. As he sends them outward, since the stream of breath is in a certain state of vibration because of the thought element permeating it, the gestures are transformed into audible speech sounds. These audible speech sounds originate in the head.

The human head has this important characteristic, that it holds itself still while the rest of the organism is built for movement and mobility. Just as a person sits still in a moving train or carriage while the horse or the carriage wheels move, so man—to the extent that he is not head—is a kind of carriage, a kind of organism for movement, and his head sits motionless on top of it all. Everything a man experiences in his head is movement of that other part of his organism that has been brought to rest. Modern physiology knows this in an external way, but only in relation to speech. It knows that there is a connection between right-hand gesturing, that is, movements of the right arm and hand, and the speech center in the left hemisphere of the brain. If one is not an outright phlegmatic, one always accompanies one's talk with gestures—northern people less, southern people more—and what one expresses by gestures comes to rest, is stopped and fixed in stillness by one's speech.

If I may turn today more particularly to those in the audience who are acquainted to some degree with anthroposophy, or who are anthroposophists, I would like to say the following. Speech has its impulse from the human head, from organs that are directed by the head. Even if some of the organs are not in the head, they nevertheless receive their impulse from it. Speech is movement that has been transformed into stillness, into fixed position by those organs. Speech is chiefly an expression of the human ego, and insofar as it is an expression of the ego, it is in constant danger of being egoistic, of being something through which the human being wants only to bring his wishes and appetites more or less to expression. If man were not restrained to some degree by his whole experience of speech in relation to his organism, he would only give expression to his inner experiences, as is the case with a child in the first primitive stages of speech when only inner emotions, impulses of will or of feeling can find expression. But as a man among men he is impelled to place himself through his speech into his whole environment. Speech is thereby given a general character and is torn away from the individual ego; it becomes the common property of a folk, of an entire human group. The fact that we do get away from the natural sounds that only bring egoistic tendencies to expression, and do adjust ourselves to the speech rooted in our folk genius, shows that there is a constant striving away from the egoistic element. This very effort, however, to work away from the egoistic state to a common element has its darker side, which the poet put so beautifully into words: "When the soul *speaks*, alas! the *soul* speaks no longer!" It is none other than the soul speaking when a child begins in his inarticulate way to

69

express what he is experiencing inwardly, even though it is merely instincts and desires. Finding himself later in unegotistical speech, in a human community with speech as its common ground, spiritualizes him for his earthly life. The soul element is spiritualized by speech.

When we accompany our speech with gestures in mime, we take what is ego activity in our speech and push it back again into our astral body, into our soul. One should try to feel what is happening there, how a person who accompanies his words with gestures—words that, naturally, he must take from the common language—obviously needs to bring some of his own personality, something individual, into the common speech. Gestures push speech back again into the soul, that is, into the astral body, into the personal.

But one feels for this reason a kind of shame toward the gestures—except for those that simply accompany ordinary speech in general—a feeling of shame because what they express belongs so particularly to one's individual personality. A person lays bare his soul, so to say, through his gestures. So when one turns to mime—this holds good as one element of dramatic art—it means that what had become more spiritual in speech is now pushed back again into the soul, into the individual human being.

Consider another way that man reveals his nature. At the head pole he reveals himself through speech, while at the foot pole, the leg pole, he reveals himself through dance.

If dance is to be really beautiful, the dancer must no longer be sticking his own egoism into it. It must be a total rhythmic offering. It must, so to say, have had all human aspects stripped away from it. When someone dances with spirit (*Schwung*), the spectator has a perception of the rhythm itself as an objective thing moving as the sweep of the music directs it (*Schwunglinie*). In dance, the human being is no longer contained within himself; he is carried out of himself completely. His body has become entirely body;

it dances among other bodies and makes movements as if there were no soul in it. What one likes in dance is the verve (*Schwung*) and the perfection of the sweep of movement (*Tanzlinie*). If the poet said, "When the soul *speaks*, alas, the *soul* speaks no longer," then for dance one should say, "When the body dances, alas, the soul is no longer there." In dance, the soul is stripped away. Speech lives in the ego; mime pushes the general content of speech into the astral body. In a similar way, dance lives in the physical body and when it is pushed into the etheric body, that is eurythmy. Eurythmy is the pushing back of the body movements of gymnastics or of dance out of their purely physical, bodily sphere back into the etheric body, which is something that stands near to the soul. Movements are given a soul content again by the eurythmist. In eurythmy, human movement in the physical world is pushed back into the spiritual, etheric world. The movement is ensouled, and if eurythmy is done properly, everything—whether single movements or group movements—is drawn from the inherent nature of man. The movements have the same lawful origin as all the speech sounds—A, I, L, M, and so on—that rise out of the human organism. In eurythmy one expresses oneself visibly through movements precisely as in speech one expresses oneself audibly through speech sounds. An A and an E are absolutely specific sounds in the area of human hearing, and any eurythmy movement is just as specific an expression in the area of the whole human being, since the eurythmy movement originates in the etheric body, the inner being of man.

One might say that in his everyday speech man expresses himself as earthly man. In the movements that are intimately related to his etheric body and that become visible speech when he does eurythmy, he reveals what the gods wanted him to be: not an earthly man but a wholly divine man who has a dwelling place in the human form. So when we look at eurythmy, we are no longer just enjoying the sweep of a

71

dance form (*Tanzschwunglinie*) and the rhythm of dance movements, but we are receiving what is said to us by cosmic man, man ensouled by the spirit—who does have something to say! If, therefore, a poem is recited or declaimed, or a piece of music is played, and eurythmy accompanies it, that is really like an orchestral ensemble.

Artistic feeling and perception are all one needs to give one a simple impression of what is happening on the stage. If usually a few words of introduction are offered, they are only for the purpose of pointing out that what appears before the audience in complete simplicity is drawn from the whole being of man, yes, from his cosmic stature. What is seemingly simple is in fact drawn from the most profound secrets of man's soul life as he lives in this world. Nothing is loftier or wiser than the unconscious utterances of a tiny child. In eurythmy, the wisdom has been drawn out more or less consciously, but this makes no difference for the immediate artistic impression.

There is no basis, therefore, for the idea that eurythmy has some sort of intellectual background. Just as in mime what originates in the head is pushed from the head down into the arms, so in eurythmy the invisible movements from within the human being are pushed up into the movement of the arms. Then one can have an impression of ensouled man, of how the whole man expresses himself in the world through his truly human nature.

All this, of course, makes it necessary that the speech artists reciting for the eurythmy shall be aware that every real poet has a certain hidden eurythmy in the way he shapes his language, in what one can call the imaginative, musical element of his language, a eurythmy that steals its way through the poet's language and lies hidden within it. That is what one must hear if one recites and declaims for eurythmy. This is not liked today; our time is too inartistic for it. Frau Dr. Steiner has worked for years to develop a style of recitation that returns to the really artistic foundation of speech. It will be through eurythmy that one finds again the eurythmic character of speech.

There are always people who come and say, "Yes, I know, we've been told that eurythmy is visible speech, that it is not dance, not mime. But what we liked best in the performance"—and again it is not the simple person speaking but the intellectual who has spent a great deal of thought on how the arts are evolving—"what we liked best were the pieces that were danced to music." Dear friends, nothing was danced to music! Just because there is music, people believe that it was danced to by the eurythmist. Things are looked at so carelessly today! In eurythmy, the music is not danced to, it is sung to—in movement. It is song-in-movement. As eurythmy is chiefly movement and speech is chiefly song, what you see accompanying the music is not dance, but singing-in-movement. One must feel this distinction as one looks at it; then one can entertain a correct judgment about it.

An understanding must gradually come about for the importance of eurythmy as an art created from artistic sources that today are still unfamiliar. An understanding will have to come for the significance of eurythmy developing in the midst of dance, mime and speech.

True speech is drawn out of human movement but not up as far as the head. If it is drawn up to the head, it becomes everyday language. If it is kept down in the arms and hands, which lie between the two poles, head and feet, there can then be expressed without slipping, I would like to say, into one extreme or the other, the real nature of man as he stands on the earth. One may also say that in speech alone, temporal man expresses what he feels about things. In eurythmy, eternal man expresses through movements what he experiences in any happening. Although eurythmy is still today in its infancy and therefore still imperfect—we know that quite well because we are our own severest critics —it will evolve further. Its medium is man himself, who is a small world containing all the secrets of the large world. Eurythmy will evolve further and will someday take its place as a fully recognized art by the side of the older arts.

# XIII

Ever since we started these eurythmy programs, I have been describing eurythmy with a few remarks. Today, I would like to speak about it from still another point of view. Eurythmy is an attempt to create a visible speech in such a living form that it will be able to reveal the experiences of the human soul more vividly and therefore more artistically than tone and speech themselves can reveal them. To realize that this is possible, one has to investigate in an honest spiritual scientific manner the process of speech formation and speech development and find how it is rooted in the human being.

Speech is, first of all, a human being's expression of what he brings out of the depths of his soul to communicate to his fellow human beings. He has physical organs to accomplish this. When one thinks about speech and song from this point of view, one can see that song offers a more differentiated expression of human soul life than speech, that is, than the speech of our civilized languages. Speech imprints some particular meaning on a tone and the tone thereby becomes a speech sound. A speech sound is a tone that contains meaning and also value. But because meaning and value—in other words, thought—has entered the sound, speech has received an inartistic element. The term "artistic" can only be applied to something that offers an image of human experience for immediate perception. One can see that song is the more artistic the more it succeeds in eliminating the importance of words and gets back to the formation of musical tone. With language, a poet must work to overcome the intellectual element by which speech serves merely for communication from man to man, the element through which it expresses abstract thought and meaning. If he would be a real poet, he must be willing to try to reveal soul experiences either by an imaginative play of his language, making one sound brighten another, a sound illuminate or darken itself, and the like, or by a musical play of language, making rhymes and alliterations, using rhythms and beat, creating motifs that are like melodies.

From this point of view, of all the poetry that is poured out into the world today in this rather inartistic time, the smallest amount can be called real poetry. Most of it is not poetry at all. A poet is not called upon to make poems about the spirit. Rather, he should be letting the spirit flow into his language; he should be seeking its revelation in the color, in the musical quality of his language.

Now one can get down to the fundamental elements of speech if one observes with spiritual scientific thinking that speech as we normally use it in the present age is altogether dependent upon the development of our nerve-sense system. Everything that our nerve-sense system experiences, flows into our breath formation, which then becomes a kind of air gesture, a gesture made of air. Just as in ordinary life, when we feel our speech is inadequate, we already help it along with gestures that can be really expressive, so in speech, "gestures" are being formed, invisible ones, in the air that is pushed out on our breath, gestures made of air. They transmit what we then hear as speech. But in these air gestures there lives and weaves and moves thought, the abstract expression of our soul life.

But now one can express what the soul experiences in quite another way. Our nerve-sense system is, after all, only one pole of our human organism. Its opposite pole is our system of movement (*Bewegungssystem*) with all that belongs

76

to it. Obviously, by means of our ordinary gestures and posture this pole of the movement system supports and reinforces those air gestures that we have found to be influenced by the nerve-sense system. But this primitive aid to our speech that our everyday gestures provide can be evolved further. We can find gestures artistically formed, clearly articulated, that relate to the ordinary gestures in the same way that articulate, beautifully perfected speech relates to the babble of a child. One can say that the gestures one sees in daily life are a kind of babbling as compared to what will come about through eurythmy as cultivated, perfectly articulated, highly developed gesture-speech.

What, then, will this accomplish? As the human being comes down from pre-earthly existence into earthly life, he becomes a citizen of the earth precisely through possessing the special equipment of a nerve-sense system that has its center in the head. It is the head that he forms first when he comes to earth, and his head is really there so that what aspires in him to have a part in physical earthly life is able to insert itself in the right way. The head sits above the rest of his physical organism so that gravity, the force coming from the earth, will be restricted in its influence. The head is not really subject to gravity; it wants to be an expression of the cosmos it resembles. Indeed, one can say that the human head shows by its form that it is born out of the cosmos where there is no gravity, and inserts itself into the active force of gravity that is controlling the human body from birth to death.

The fact that the human being learns an earthly language and sings earthly words to his music, means that he is subject to a certain degree to the force of gravity coming from the earth. He is subject to it most of all in his movement system. When he walks, when he moves his hands and arms, gravity is continually active in these movements. He overcomes its force to some extent since, with every step he takes, the free, weightless part of his organism is fighting the gravity that is weighing him down and that is weighing all human beings down during earthly life.

Now one is privileged to see something quite beautiful when an action takes place that, in a definite sense, does underlie speech; that is, when the weightless, superearthly human being enters the realm of gravity and overcomes the earthly force that normally permeates our movement organism. It is this force from which every step, every hand and arm gesture has tried continually, unconsciously and weakly to free itself. Now a song is "sung," for instance, simply by rhythmic movements. Our most expressive human movements, those of hands and arms, are transformed from gestures weighed down by gravity into free gestures. Now one sees something highly important: the human being, even as he stands there within the sphere of gravity, overcomes the force by means of his own soul forces.

Thus, while the ordinary speech we use as we stand within gravity has become an instrument for abstract expression, the endeavor of eurythmy to overcome gravity by living gestures of hands and arms becomes a new kind of speech that accomplishes the exact opposite. Our ordinary speech carries heaven down to earth and, as it were, fits heaven into earth. Eurythmy, however, creates its gesture-speech by its conscious overcoming of gravity in the movement system; it enables a human being to pull away from the earth and express the life of his soul in such a way that with every gesture he seems to assert: I carry a heavenly man within my earthly man.

If one would express it a little more imaginatively, one could say that with the ordinary indifferent gestures by which we reinforce our everyday earthly speech, there are angelic beings standing by and helping. If these everyday gestures are then transformed into the articulate gestures of eurythmy, into a speech that flows from one being to another, then what one sees is actually what the archangels are saying to one another.

Man thus raises himself from hard ground to a realm where divine spiritual beings are communicating in the special way that is characteristic of them, where movements, one might say, are not restrained by force of gravity but are free to sweep unhindered through cosmic space. Not to be caught in gravity means to be reaching toward eternity. So eurythmy liberates the eternal man in earthly man. The divine spiritual being that dwells in all men comes to expression through temporal earthly man. When the human soul engages itself with eurythmy, it seems to pour itself into the transient human form out of the eternal wellspring of human nature.

Something is thereby created that gives essential support to the art of recitation and declamation. The poet has already striven to overcome the earthly character of his language by grasping its musical, rhythmic elements. In recitation it is above all the eurythmic qualities that must be sought, as Frau Dr. Steiner has been endeavoring to do for years. It is not the abstract content of the poems that should be emphasized but the structure of the language, the musical, sculptural, artistic elements. Then, when music or recitation are accompanied by eurythmy, that is, by the living force of a human being as he overcomes gravity, pushing gravity away, as it were, by the spirited movements of his limbs, then we have an orchestral collaboration that can bring to expression all the inner artistic beauty of the poem, of the song, or of the music in a way that otherwise is not at all possible.

After all, there are tremendous depths to real art. Now, when I make such a remark, I must at once beg you, dear friends, to be charitable! While we are setting ourselves distant goals, we realize that we are only at the beginning of the course. We are our own severest critics. But we know that

79

eurythmy holds endless possibilities of development. It frees the higher human being from gravity so that he is able to reveal his divine spiritual nature. One can hope, therefore, that eurythmy will develop further and further until it is finally an art as fully recognized as the other arts that have long since won recognition. This may take a long time, but there should be an ever-increasing interest in the early stages of our endeavor to create this new art form.

# XIV

To grasp the full significance of eurythmy, one must realize that it is an attempt to create an actual visible speech and an actual visible song, so that music that is being played or poetry that is being recited can be presented at the same time on the stage in visible form.

First of all, one must realize that every human manifestation in the physical world comes out of the totality of our human nature. Yet, we really have nothing more in complete waking consciousness than our ideas, our concepts. We do not experience our feelings to the same degree of wakefulness as we do our ideas. Our feelings are only at the level of dream consciousness. Only to the extent that we have transformed them into ideas have they become awake. Our life of will is completely submerged in sleep; indeed, in dreamless sleep. It is pushed down to the level of total unconsciousness. Of our will impulses we only experience whatever thought element may be contained in them. We get an idea to make some movement; the idea disappears into our organism and we know nothing of it until we move. The intention that starts our willing, and then the action that we perform, are present as ideas in our waking consciousness. What goes on within us in order to bring the will impulse into action is as completely enveloped in sleep as our entire soul life is enveloped in sleep between the moment of falling asleep and awakening.

But now, when we express ourselves in speech or song, we are creating something out of our whole human nature.

Let us consider speech first. When we speak a sentence, our whole being is revealed in it. Our feeling, which normally we experience at dream level, is now the thread weaving through the words, through the sounds. Likewise, our impulse of will works its way into the words, into the sounds. But, leaving aside such abnormal phenomena as talking in one's sleep, we have to be fully awake when we speak. Thus, even so, there is an unconscious element rising from the depth of our being that shows itself in the way our words are uttered, by the sounds coming out strong or weak, and so forth.

As we speak in normal daily life, we adjust ourselves to every kind of circumstance and we let thought predominate in our words. But thought is an inartistic element. An artistic quality can only begin to be present in speech when thought is no longer active, and I mean, not only the thought exercised in imparting knowledge, but even the thought that is conveyed from man to man in everyday conventional life. Thought activity as such is inartistic.

A poet has to deal with thoughts because—well, for the simple reason that language must provide a place where thoughts can live! But a poet's chief task is to take what he hears sounding from the unconscious levels of his being and weave this into his language, making the language imaginative and musical. From a poet's point of view, language only has an artistic quality if it is pliant so that it can be molded, if the speech sounds are given imaginative color, if the phrases are given a musical quality, if rhythms and meter are delicately worked out. Thus, the poet must give his thought content a form by working the unconscious elements into it. He must let a feeling element and will element stream into it. One cannot have them stream into one's normal thinking because thinking is something alien to both elements. But the poet can let them stream through his work as he molds his language.

When I say, "The tree is becoming green" (*Der Baum grünt*), I have first of all expressed a thought and my language is dry and abstract. But the moment I depart from conventional usage and say, "The greening tree" (*grünender Baum*), I have already infused a nuance of feeling into my language. I can increase this by accelerating the beat, changing the rhythm, and so forth. By varying the stress, I can give more play to the will element that is also streaming into my language.

So a poet's language has eurythmy hidden in it that originates in his feeling and will. This is what the speech artist must work particularly to reveal. Otherwise, he is only giving a prose reading, not a real recitation or declamation such as Frau Dr. Steiner has for years been developing here. Only if the speech artist gives his recitation or declamation a truly eurythmic character, can true eurythmy be performed by the eurythmist.

It is possible with spiritual scientific perception to observe what flows from the unconscious into speech and song. One can observe, for instance, what the feeling element is in any spoken phrase, and also what the will element is. When someone speaks, this is all pushed up to his head and his thought is colored or given a musical quality. One can trace back and discover how the feeling and will colored his thought, affected its shape and made it musical. It came about through his movement system (*Bewegungssystem*). One can therefore represent it by movements and gestures that will themselves be made by a human being, that will themselves come from the human movement system. As a person makes these movements, there is first of all a spatial element to be found in them: it is, if you look for it in human speech, the imaginative activity that goes into the shaping of each sound. There is also a time element: that is, the way one movement follows another, the way they are coordinated and harmonized, the way they make a kind of melody. This time element can even be made into melodic themes. It is precisely the musical element in language that shows us how language is grounded in the human movement system. You can make a melody out of the way a man walks, or you can tap out a rhythm; you can even hum a so-called "musical embellishment" from the way he moves! In other words, everything that declamation should be concerned with is obtained from one's observation of the unconscious impulses in human movement; it is certainly not to be found in human thoughts. All this is to be seen in specific eurythmy gestures and spatial eurythmy movements.

So an art form has been created that is neither dance nor mere gesture. Everyday gestures are really a kind of eurythmic baby-talk that help us out when we are unable to express something in words of abstract thought. If we're fellows without a speck of temperament, we stick our hands in our pockets and manage somehow without gestures; but some of us have feelings and our hands itch to make gestures. Such gestures relate to eurythmy as a child's babbling relates to articulate speech. In eurythmy, a gesture does not merely point to the existence of some feeling or other; the gesture itself contains the feeling in the shape it makes, the shape that is there immediately in space or that unfolds in a time sequence. Thereby, what in the everyday gesture is only an unconscious hint is in eurythmy transformed into direct perception. When someone makes ordinary gestures, we notice them and feel them rather unconsciously. But the movements made in eurythmy are really to be looked at with watchful eyes. Something is being displayed before our physical senses for our physical perception that usually, when someone speaks or sings, takes place at the subconscious level, only revealing itself through his temperament, through the sound of his voice or the color of his tone. Eurythmy is a visible art in the most eminent sense. If one has the idea that he has to exercise some kind of intellectual activity while looking at it, then one is misjudging it. One doesn't have to analyze those forms (*Formen*) that the eurythmist follows. One should simply enjoy them artistically, esthetically, feel a healthy joy watching them. Everything one can think up to say about eurythmy in abstract words is really only artificial. The real content of eurythmy is the spatial forms that one sees and the sequence of movements in time. That is what it is all about. Eurythmy expresses the content of a poem visibly, or a piece of music visibly.

So it should become clear to us that the speech we learn as children and use until the end of our life, is only something for our earth life. It is foolish to believe, as spiritualism does, that departed souls use ordinary human speech. They no longer have a national language; they have worked their way out of it. When they died they ceased being English, French, Italian, and so forth. They have simply entered another sphere. Therefore, it makes no sense to believe that the dead can accomplish some immediate materialization in a specific language. What they say must first be translated into human speech. Speech is a product of earth life and is fitted to earthly conditions. If a man longs in the depths of his soul to make his speech less earthly, he takes to gestures. The reverse is also true: A man who likes to stand as stiff as a poker and talk as stiff as a poker is always, if not in his world outlook, surely in his feelings, materialistic, earthy. Someone who speaks more out of the spiritual world is always impelled to accompany his conversation with gestures, because what is expressed by our ordinary gestures has meaning in the spiritual sphere immediately adjoining our world. There our gestures are experienced as speech. It is as if beings from the angelic world, the world of the Angeloi, were always encouraging us to strengthen our earth speech with the help from supersensible realms.

85

But now, if we consider eurythmy, if we examine the gestures in the visible speech of eurythmy, we find that they place us in the realm of the archangels—of course, in a certain sense, unconsciously, and more so or less so; when one undertakes to create eurythmy, for instance, it must be done out of an absolutely clear consciousness. We find that our eurythmy movements are speech in the realm of the archangels. So we are providing a significant superearthly element as accompaniment for the poet's creation, which he, on his part, has worked to raise to a superearthly level by rejecting its prose character and, instead, infusing into it color, form and music.

Of course, it may sound rather fantastic when one says that eurythmy is the earthly image of the speech of the archangels. But however it may sound, for someone whose thoughts are not materialistic it is actually true! When the poet says, "When the soul *speaks*, alas! the *soul* is speaking no longer," he is right, because he feels that something deserving to be given artistic form is in every instance degraded when it is thrown into prose language. It must first be lifted out by the art of recitation and declamation, which restores poetic qualities to the art of poetry. What the poet experiences, what does not belong to the sense world, can be expressed precisely through these movements in eurythmic language. Every art, in fact, raises what is of the earth to a view of heaven; this is known to everyone who has lived in a really artistic atmosphere. It remained for this present epoch of materialism no longer to feel joy when it looks at Raphael's pictures. I experienced this with many artists I knew at the turn of the century. His pictures were too unearthly for them. They preferred to paint the warts on a man's face so as to have as much earthiness in their pictures as possible. One of them even told me—it was someone whose painting in earlier years had been especially valued by the theosophists—that he was the first artist to have the courage to put hair on his nudes wherever a person normally has hair. While the other artists were willing to ignore such complete earthiness, he considered it especially clever. Michelangelo? Such people said, "Well, today he is still accepted since he at least tried to come down to earth." But Raphael? For many of them, he was impossible to swallow!

But every art wants to enhance the things of earth with a superearthly sheen. Actually, art only has its true justification if it does so.

So one may say that eurythmy, developing a new art form from the smallest beginning, is opening up a new path; such paths have always been opened up as genuine art forms have arisen in the evolution of mankind. One may therefore wish this new art a full life because it does not disavow its true spiritual origin—the origin of every fine art. This makes its future unquestionably assured.

# XV*

At our last eurythmy performance the day before yesterday, I made a few remarks concerning the relation of what one might call this moving sculpture, eurythmy, to our ordinary motionless sculpture. Eurythmy is an art that has to do with the moving human being; it uses movements that have been found within the human organism and brought out as a kind of speech. With eurythmy a new art form has appeared that can be broadened and developed in the most manifold ways, and as it gradually unfolds it can be connected with the other arts, even confronting them with this or that significant contrast.

I have pointed out that in eurythmy one sees moving sculpture. Eurythmy can also be described in another way. If one considers the arts that are most closely associated with human speech, one realizes that, in contrast to speech, music and song must be thought of as reaching into the inner life of a human being. When the human soul gives itself up to the melodies and harmonies of music, the importance of this musical involvement lies in the fact that music does not relate to anything so definitely as does speech. One can even say that when one turns from musical activity to speech activity it is, in a sense, a process of waking up. When someone speaks, he feels awake as compared to his feeling when he is musically involved.

---

*During the Christmas conference at the Goetheanum. GA 260

It cannot be denied, however, that waking and sleeping are relative concepts. One who has formerly had no experience of the spiritual world, but who gradually gains such a connection, feels at first that, compared to daily life, experience of the spiritual world is like sleeping. If, however, someone maintains complete awareness as he goes from ordinary day consciousness into the other world, he experiences, in what for the other person is sleep, actually a higher level of wakefulness. One can also say that when someone begins to experience the broader, cosmic significance of music as compared to speech, he can regard this experience likewise as an awakening. One can think of a melody being more and more compressed and squeezed together in time. Then, finally, through the intensity of the compression a vowel or a consonant can actually result. Then the music that lies inherent in the speech sound is no longer perceived; the speech sound is in reality a melodic or harmonic element that has been compressed. Just as one can feel this objectively about the relation of music to speech, one can also express it by saying that music is nearer to human feeling, while poetry is nearer to human imagination. The imagery of poetry is to be found in the various elements of speech.

One can also raise perception itself. The senses that do the perceiving lie still farther outside than imagination—that is, at the very periphery—and this can also be raised to an artistic level. In music one lives in a sea of flowing spirit, as it were. In speech it is as if one had reached the shore of this spirit sea. Imagination is what lives on the shore between water and earth. Now, when one comes out of the water and gives oneself entirely to the sensory world, at the same time perceiving the spirit in it, one reaches something that does not become speech but can only be represented by signs that originate within oneself. One reaches eurythmy.

Deep within us an artistic, musical activity weaves and

shapes our feeling world. Somewhat nearer to the periphery a poetic activity shapes our world of ideas into artistic language. Beyond the periphery, outside our world of ideas, we have already gone out of ourselves and live in perception. What we experience in perception, not physically but spiritually, is what eurythmy contains.

Actually, when one is watching eurythmy, one ought to be able to sniff nature in all of it, and surmise the spirit in all of nature. Whoever does so is perceiving eurythmy in the right way. One can imagine that someone seeing eurythmy could say: That eurythmy movement reminds me of an impression I had the other day when I was walking through the woods, of a fir tree swaying in the wind. If he does not simply keep to this feeling but later is able to say: Yes, eurythmy has finally given me an explanation of that fir tree; it is not standing there just to be a fir tree; it is one letter in the eternal Word that surges and weaves through the world; eurythmy explains to me how the fir tree speaks, how the brook speaks, how the lightning speaks, and so on and so on.—When someone can say this, he has observed eurythmy in the right way.

This present age only uses the word "explanation" for what is given to one in the form of ideas or abstract concepts. But Nature is not so poor or so horribly grey as our abstract concepts. One had better watch out if he thinks he has got firm hold of Nature simply by forcing her into his web of concepts in which he thinks he can describe her. Nature is endlessly rich, not merely in extent but in depth, not merely in quantity but in quality. If we want to come close to her, we must make a much stronger effort than by simply using our heads. Our heads know little about a fir tree. We have to awaken our fantasy, every bit of fantasy that is in us, if we want to describe lovingly and out of our own humanity the secrets of spiritual Nature that are in every single thing and in every single process. Only when

91

we are able to create something out of Nature that then arouses in us a feeling of awe for what the World-All has formed through us, with us, in us—only then have we attained a really artistic level, the level at which every art in the history of the world has been born. Indeed, it is only at such a level that we will be able to accomplish the proper development of this new art, eurythmy.

Particularly where anthroposophy is being cultivated, there should be serious concern that artistic work—especially a new artistic endeavor such as eurythmy—will be received and understood with warm sympathy. In recent times art has suffered considerably because people only value the knowledge they acquire from dull, dry concepts. So art has gradually become a luxury of life. If this continues, a frightful philistinism will be spread over the earth. Humanity will inevitably have a benighted future unless really fresh new art is created from artistic sources still untapped. That is what we have tried to do here in our own field of work with eurythmy. One so longs to find a right feeling for the artistic importance of this new art in the Anthroposophical Society!

But one has to realize that art is creative out of its very being, and that one falls short of art the moment one begins to "illustrate." You can have poetry that is recited or declaimed in the proper style accompanied by eurythmy; they belong together: eurythmy, in which the whole human organism is involved in movement, and recitation or declamation, concentrated for their delivery in a particular group of organs. Both of these arts will develop independently. But they will work together as heart and head work together in the human organism because, although they are quite different from each other, they are organized for each other.

Eurythmy accompanies instrumental music, of course, that is played on some instrument separate from the player. But you cannot do eurythmy to singing! If you did, you would only be illustrating the song through its musical content, which is something decidedly inartistic. Mere illustration is definitely inartistic. Perhaps some day, in addition to the song or, if you will, the song accompanied by an instrument, one will also want to perform eurythmy, but it will have to be something entirely different from our present tone eurythmy and speech eurythmy. Certainly the arts can work together, but because the wish has been expressed to do eurythmy to singing, I am obliged to speak of it. If a person really understands that in our tone eurythmy there is already singing by the movements themselves, that eurythmy is itself singing to this or that instrument or even to the orchestra, then that person will not want the singing to be doubled! That is the whole point of the matter.

# XVI

May I say a few words to introduce our eurythmy performance? Certainly not to "explain" it! It would not be my
idea to explain art either in general or in special performances. But perhaps I may tell you about the artistic sources
from which eurythmy has been created, which today are
still unfamiliar, and of the medium that eurythmy uses.

You will see that a eurythmy performance consists of one
or more individuals moving in space. At first glance, it may
seem to be an art of gestures, but it is not that. Or it may
look like a new dance art; it is not that either. Eurythmy is
actually visible speech raised to the level of art by virtue of
its very special character. Speech itself, of course, must also
be raised to the same level. Eurythmy can be called "visible
song" when it accompanies instrumental music.

When a human being speaks, he is pouring into sounds
what he experiences in his soul; the sounds are forming into
words, the words into sentences, and so on. Finally, a poet's
artistic handling of all this creates something that has
rhythm and beat with pictorial and sculptural qualities. One
should realize that every single speech sound takes a definite
shape and has its own particular form in the air that the
speaker exhales. The form is brought about by the combined activity of larynx, palate, tongue, lips, etc.

What thus issues forth from the human being and reaches
to his fellowmen, what has been metamorphosed into speech
and language, has had its origin in the entire human organism. Today, except for one small detail, there is little

95

knowledge of this fact. It is generally known that in most people the speech center, that is, the organ from which comes the impulse to speak, is on the left side of the brain. But this is not always the case. In a few people it is on the right side. These are the "left-handers." The fact that "normal," right-handed people, who always perform certain activities with their right hands, have their speech center on the left side of the brain, naturally means nothing until one learns that the left-handed people have their speech center on the right side. One is then obliged to see a connection between speech and the movements of arms and hands.

Just think what this implies for the most expressive of our bodily organs, the arms and hands! Our soul stirs within us so strongly when we are especially moved that we feel impelled to accompany our words with gestures; that is, to pour our feeling directly and at the same time into arm and hand movements. Often one finds one can understand someone better from his gestures than from his language! In many people this speech of their hands and arms can be most expressive. Particularly in civilized languages there is such a conventional content, and also such detail of abstract knowledge that Schiller's verse can be applied literally: "When the soul *speaks*, alas, the *soul* speaks no longer!" We adjust our speech to conventional or to intellectual constraints, but we disclose much more of our individuality when we make use of a gesture.

As with our arms, so, too, we can make gestures with other parts of our body. But all this kind of gesturing is as far removed from what eurythmy is intended to be as a child's babbling is removed from articulated, cultivated speech. To someone who inquires deeply into the nature of the human being, what goes into speech—what eventually are air gestures through which the speech sounds are conveyed—what goes into speech depends originally on what the entire human being wants to express through gestures. One has here a fragment of knowledge of the connection that exists between definite inclinations to movement that are present in the human organism and the final production of speech through the speech center in the brain. Anthroposophy has knowledge of this connection; it is anthroposophy, therefore, that can open up wider horizons.

When we have something to say, there is usually something about it that we want to stress. We stress one word particularly if we want to emphasize something, while another word we will stress less. So we proceed through all the levels from light to heavy emphasis. This is not so much connected with our impulse to make arm gestures as it is with the way we show our personality in our walking. Whoever has a sense for these things knows exactly from the way someone walks—whether more strongly, for instance, on the ball of his foot or on his heels—just how he will stress this or that in his speech.

One can also observe someone's speech from the point of view of grammar. This has to do with the thought element, which is the most inartistic element of speech. If our intellect predominates in the forming of our speech, then what we want to express by gestures will be accomplished primarily through head movements. If, for instance, some boring know-it-all wants to show you that he takes great care in arriving at his judgments, he will make this gesture [Dr. Steiner demonstrates], or he will lay a finger on his nose, or take hold of his nose. That shows the head dominance.

But all that lies between intellect and will (emphasis in speech comes from the will), what lies between in the realm of feeling, what the poet pours into rhythm and rhyme, into his choice of meters, and so forth—this is the really artistic element of speech. It can come to expression quite naturally through movements of the arms and hands, supported by a person's other movements. Dance emphasizes the will ele-

97

ment, mime the intellectual; the real feeling element is expressed by eurythmy.

The poet felt quite rightly that the human soul is no longer to be found in speech. But speech can be brought back again into gestures. What a child really wants to put into gestures is unconsciously concentrated in his speech organ. If one now gives that back again to the impulses toward movement of the whole human organism, one then has created a visible speech. The single movements relate to single speech sounds. A sequence of movements has the same significance as our customary sequences of sounds, sentence connections, and so forth, in our everyday speech. Eurythmy is in very truth visible speech. It can also become visible song.

As visible speech, eurythmy is accompanied here by recitation and declamation. Their collaboration shows at once that in its treatment of a poem eurythmy is involved completely with the artistic content. Today, in our inartistic age, there is no proper understanding for our attitude. People are only interested in emphasizing the prose content of a poem, but that has no value! One must look to the poet's style, to something that is being expressed on a higher level than prose, something that works its way into the poem through the musical element or the pictorial, through the sculptural, the color elements of the poet's language. Recitation and declamation must be brought back to what they were at the time when Goethe rehearsed his iambic dramas with his actors with a baton in hand like a choral conductor. He did that because he knew that the essential quality of language lies in its musical and imaginative elements. The feeling in a poem has quite a different power when, for instance, the reciter puts variety into the beat or rhythm of his recitation, than it does when it is merely expressed in the prose content. That is why the "secret eurythmy" already hidden in the poet's language must be of foremost interest when recitation and declamation accompany the eurythmy.

Unfamiliar as eurythmy still is today, so equally unfamiliar is this art of recitation and declamation that pays more attention to the style of the language than to the prose content. One hopes that eurythmy will help to create an understanding for what the art should be. One can feel what eurythmy is intended to be when one sees it as visible song accompanying instrumental music. If a person were to sing and at the same time perform eurythmy gestures for the words or for the notes of the song, you would at once have the feeling that there is something wrong there! Whoever would do this has not really understood the nature of eurythmy. It would be the same as if a person were singing a solo and someone else stood up to sing, too. There must be the feeling that a eurythmist is not dancing to the music but singing to it, singing with her arms. Once one has felt this difference between dance and the tone eurythmy that is presented here, one has really grasped the nature of eurythmy. This can, after all, only be understood through feeling.

But you will say: I suppose one has first to study eurythmy to find out what all those movements mean. That is not necessary. It is only important that the movements and their sequences make an artistic impression. Eurythmy must create its effect through immediate artistic perception, and it will truly have this effect. As you watch it accompanying the recitation of a poem, you will have the impression that this is the only way it could be done! There is no other way to perform eurythmy for that poem! Down to the smallest movement there is nothing arbitrary, nothing personal. It is exactly as with speech; with speech you simply cannot use any random sound in place of another. If, for instance, you want to talk about "bread," you cannot say "breed." Likewise, in eurythmy no other movement can be made than the one that corresponds to the speech sound the reciter is uttering.

So eurythmy becomes a moving sculpture. One has the feeling that our customary motionless sculpture portrays the silent human soul in all its stillness. A soul that is surging and struggling to speak can only be portrayed by bringing the living human form into movement. From this point of view, eurythmy is moving sculpture.

Dear friends, we well know that our eurythmy is at its most rudimentary stage. We ourselves are our severest critics! There will be more and more performances here, there and everywhere with a rich variety of programs; we expect them to be criticized, especially by the professional critics. We believe that we know better than anyone else all the justified criticisms of this beginning we have made. We know that it is far from perfect. Even so, we are confident that it has endless possibilities of development. Since it is using the most perfect medium one could have for an art, the human being himself, all cosmic secrets and laws can be brought to expression. Man is a small world, a microcosm, that can disclose the secrets of the outer world, the macrocosm. Since eurythmy has a perfect instrument and will always have it, since the secrets of the human being in motion will be studied and artistically revealed more and more, eurythmy will undoubtedly make its way in the world. With eurythmy as with everything else, beginnings are difficult. But the artistic sources of eurythmy that today are still strange, and the artistic style that is also still strange, will be gradually understood.

# FOR FURTHER READING

Rudolf Steiner intended these carefully written volumes to serve as a foundation to all of the later, more advanced anthroposophical writings and lecture courses.

THE PHILOSOPHY OF SPIRITUAL ACTIVITY by Rudolf Steiner. "Is human action free?" asks Steiner in his most important philosophical work. By first addressing the nature of knowledge, Steiner cuts across the ancient debate of real or illusory human freedom. A painstaking examination of human experience as a polarity of percepts and concepts shows that only in thinking does one escape the compulsion of natural law. Steiner's argument arrives at the recognition of the self-sustaining, universal reality of thinking that embraces both subjective and objective validity. Free acts can be performed out of love for a "moral intuition" grasped ever anew by a living thinking activity. Steiner scrutinizes numerous world-views and philosophical positions and finally indicates the relevance of his conclusion to human relations and life's ultimate questions.

KNOWLEDGE OF THE HIGHER WORLDS AND ITS ATTAINMENT by Rudolf Steiner. Rudolf Steiner's fundamental work on the path to higher knowledge explains in detail the exercises and disciplines a student must pursue in order to attain a wakeful experience of supersensible realities. The stages of Preparation, Enlightenment, and Initiation are described, as is the transformation of dream-life and the meeting with the Guardian of the Threshold. Moral exercises for developing each of the spiritual lotus petal organs ("chakras") are given in accordance with the rule of taking three steps in moral development for each step into spiritual knowledge. The path described here is a safe one which will not interfere with the student's ability to lead a normal outer life.

THEOSOPHY, AN INTRODUCTION TO THE SUPERSENSIBLE KNOWLEDGE OF THE WORLD AND THE DESTINATION OF MAN by Rudolf Steiner. In this work Steiner carefully explains many of the basic concepts and terminologies of anthroposophy. The book begins with a sensitive description of the primordial trichotomy: body, soul, and spirit, elaborating the various higher members of the human constitution. A discussion of reincarnation and karma follows. The next and longest chapter presents, in a vast panorama, the seven regions of the soul world, the seven regions of the land of spirits, and the soul's journey after death through these worlds. A brief discussion of the path to higher knowledge follows.

AN OUTLINE OF OCCULT SCIENCE by Rudolf Steiner. This work begins with a thorough discussion and definition of the term "occult" science. A description of the supersensible nature of the human being follows, along with a discussion of dreams, sleep, death, life between death and rebirth, and reincarnation. In the fourth chapter evolution is described from the perspective of initiation science. The fifth chapter characterizes the training a student must undertake as a preparation for initiation. The sixth and seventh chapters consider the future evolution of the world and more detailed observations regarding supersensible realities.